Saw Palmetto

Saw Palmetto

NATURAL PROSTATE RELIEF

DR SARAH BREWER

Thorsons

While the author of this work has made every effort to ensure that the information contained in this book is as accurate and up to date as possible at the time of publication, medical and pharmaceutical knowledge is constantly changing and the application of it to particular circumstances depends on many factors. Therefore it is recommended that readers always consult a qualified medical specialist for individual advice. This book should not be used as an alternative to seeking specialist medical advice, which should be sought before any action is taken. The authors and publishers cannot be held responsible for any errors and omissions that may be found in the text, or any actions that may be taken by a reader as a result of any reliance on the information contained in the text, which is taken entirely at the reader's own risk.

Thorsons
An Imprint of HarperCollins*Publishers*
77–85 Fulham Palace Road,
Hammersmith, London W6 8JB
The Thorsons website address is: www.thorsons.com

Published by Thorsons 2000

10 9 8 7 6 5 4 3 2 1

A catalogue record for this book
is available from the British Library

ISBN 0 7225 3960 6

Printed in Great Britain by
Woolnough Bookbinding Ltd, Irthlingborough, Northants

Contents

SAW PALMETTO

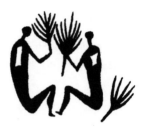

Saw Palmetto

NATURAL PROSTATE RELIEF

Introduction:

Natural Treatments for Prostate Problems

Interest in natural treatments for prostate problems has increased dramatically in recent years. As a result, Saw Palmetto (botanical names *Serenoa repens, Sabal serrulata*) is now one of the most widely-prescribed remedies for prostate problems in Continental Europe. In Germany and Austria, herbal extracts are used as first-line treatment for men with benign prostatic hyperplasia (BPH) and account for over 90 per cent of all drugs prescribed to treat BPH.[1] In Italy, plant extracts represent almost 50 per cent of treatments for BPH, while synthetic drugs such as alpha-blockers and 5-alpha-reductase inhibitors account for only around 5 per cent each of BPH treatments – statistics which I find absolutely fascinating.[2]

The use of herbal extracts to treat medical problems is known as *phytotherapy*. It is both a science and an art, and in many cases is based on sound research principles. Few people realize that as many as 40 per cent of medically prescribed drugs are derived from traditional plant remedies – the most famous of these include aspirin (from the willow tree), morphine (from the opium poppy), digoxin (from the foxglove), oral contraceptive pills (originally derived from diosgenin, extracted from the Mexican yam) and even powerful new cancer treatments such as vincristine and vinblastine (from the rosy periwinkle), and paclitaxel (from the Pacific Yew Tree). Of these plant-derived drugs, modern technology can still only synthesize seven more cheaply than they can be extracted and purified from the plants themselves.[3]

Because plants are such a rich and cheap source of pharmaceutically useful substances, specialists – known as ethnobotanists – are continually seeking new products from among the traditional herbs used by native healers worldwide.

Different parts of different plants are used in phytotherapy – roots, stems, flowers, leaves, bark, sap, fruit or seeds, depending on which has the highest concentration of active ingredient. In most cases these are dried and ground to produce a powder which is made into an aqueous infusion (tea or tisane), an alcoholic solution (tincture), or packed into tablets/capsules.

Phytotherapy is widely used for treating symptoms caused by enlargement of the prostate gland – the condition known as benign prostatic hyperplasia, or BPH for short. Extracts of the fruit of the Saw Palmetto – or dwarf American palm tree – are the most widely studied of these.

Saw Palmetto has been used for centuries by Native Americans as both a nutritional male tonic and to treat a range of genito-urinary problems including underactive testicles (hypogonadism), irritation of the male genital tract, and urinary symptoms due to BPH. It has been so effective that it has often been referred to as the *plant catheter*. Saw Palmetto is also widely regarded as a pro-sexual herb, or aphrodisiac, to improve impotence and low sex drive in men.

Most importantly, no serious side-effects have been reported from the millions of doses taken.

Several other natural plant products are also used to treat BPH. These include:

- Rye pollen (*Secale cereale*)
- Evening primrose (*Oenothera biennis*)
- South African star grass (*Hypoxis rooperi*)
- Stinging nettle (*Urtica dioica, Urtica urens*)
- Pumpkin seed (*Cucurbita pepo*)
- African prune (*Pygeum africanum*)
- Evening primrose oil.

Like conventional drugs, these extracts improve prostate symptoms in a number of different ways. Some shrink or soften the gland so the urethra stays open more easily. Others relax the muscles of the prostate and bladder so that passing water is more easy.

Until recently, many doctors have questioned how effective phytotherapy is for treating BPH symptoms, and it is not unusual to see comments such as 'probably no better than placebo' littered throughout the literature. A review[4] published in 1997 helped to squash the unbelievers by showing that several new clinical studies demonstrated significant benefits for phytotherapy when compared with inactive, placebo treatments.

Based on these results, the reviewer stated that the use of phytotherapy for mild to moderate symptoms of BPH was well justified.

The trend towards herbal medicine is accompanied by a general increased interest in health, especially in healthy eating, taking vitamin and mineral supplements and following a healthier lifestyle. More and more people are taking responsibility for their own health; the information contained in this book will help men to take responsibility for their own prostate gland.

Quotes from Men with Prostate Symptoms

'The worst thing is that I can't go on any sort of travel without there being toilets.'

'Having to keep going to the loo embarrasses me considerably – I don't like spending long periods of time with anyone except my wife.'

'One of the worst aspects is not getting a proper night's sleep. I'm fed up of having to go to the bathroom a dozen times a night.'

'I have to wear a pad in my pyjamas at night to save the mattress from urinary leakage.'

'On a bad day I just dribble, dribble, dribble. It's not painful, but it is uncomfortable and I worry about the smell.'

'When I have to go, I have to go. I have to drop whatever I'm doing and hope I can reach the toilet in time.'

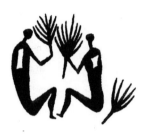

The Prostate Gland

CHAPTER ONE

Most men know more about a woman's monthly cycle than they do about their own body and its sexual health, yet problems with the prostate gland are as common in men as period problems in women. Because the gland is hidden away deep in the 'plumbing', and because it generally behaves itself until middle age, it comes as something of a shock when it starts to go wrong.

Four main problems can affect the prostate gland:

1 Benign prostatic hyperplasia, in which the gland slowly enlarges

2 Prostatitis, in which the gland becomes infected or inflamed

3 Prostatodynia, in which prostate pain occurs with no obvious cause

4 Prostate cancer.

Prostate Anatomy

The prostate is a sexual and reproductive gland that is only found in males. It lies just below the base of the bladder and is wrapped around the urethra – the tube through which urine flows from the bladder to the outside world.

At birth, the prostate gland is around the size of a pea. It slowly increases in size until puberty, when it puts on a rapid growth spurt. Between early adulthood and the age of around 40 years (when it starts to enlarge again), a healthy prostate gland weighs around 20 g and has been compared in size and shape to a large chestnut. It is made up of three anatomical parts – a median and two lateral lobes – which are separated from one another by the central urethra, two ejaculatory ducts and a fibrous band.

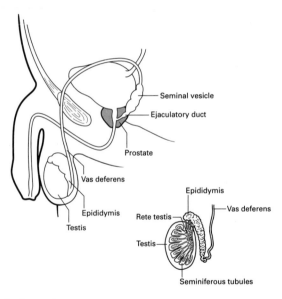

Male reproductive system

The prostate is surrounded and protected by two capsules: the true capsule – a thin, fibrous sheath – and the false capsule, which is made up of a rather flimsy tissue that is continuous with that surrounding the bladder and separates the gland from the rectum (fascia of Denonvilliers).

The prostate is made up of millions of tiny glands that secrete prostatic fluids, fibre cells that maintain its shape and structure, and muscle cells that help the gland to contract. It is not really a single gland, but is made up of millions of tiny glands separated from one another by the muscle and fibre cells. Because of this, it is sometimes referred to as the functional prostatic unit.

The Prostatic Urethra

The part of the urinary exit tube that passes through the prostate is known as the prostatic urethra. This is the widest and most dilatable part of the male urethra. It is around 3 cm long and passes down through the prostate gland in a slightly forwards direction.

The upper part of the prostatic urethra has a small raised area known as the urethral crest. At the top of this crest is a small pit, the prostatic utricle, into which the ejaculatory ducts open. The ejaculatory ducts discharge fluid from the seminal vesicles and sperm which have travelled from the testes up the vas deferens on either side. In the groove on either side of the crest up to 30 prostatic ducts discharge secretions from the prostate gland tissues.

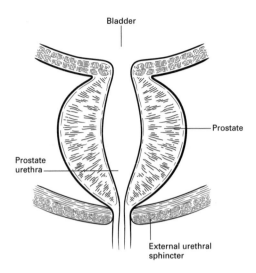

A healthy prostate

Prostate Secretions

The prostatic ducts discharge a thin, milky fluid which is acidic due to its high citric acid content. Prostatic secretions keep the lining of the urethra moist and make up around a third of semen volume. The fluid contains vitamins, minerals, amino acids and sugars which help to keep sperm healthy, but are not essential for reproduction.

Prostate enzymes such as PSA (prostate specific antigen) liquefy the clotted secretions produced by the seminal vesicles, so that sperm can swim through the semen more easily. As PSA is produced only in the prostate gland, it is a useful marker for detecting prostate cancer (see page 33).

The prostate gland is most famous as the site of the discovery of hormone-like chemicals known as prostaglandins. These are now known to exist in all tissues of the body, but those produced in the prostate are able to trigger pouting of the female cervix so sperm can gain access to the upper female tract more easily. Other components of prostatic fluid may play an immunosuppressant role to protect sperm once they are in the female environment.

Prostate Valve

The male reproductive and urinary systems are closely linked as they share the same exit tube – the urethra – which runs through the centre of the penis. One of the most important functions of the prostate is, therefore, the way it acts like a valve. It forms part of a structure known as the internal sphincter, which contracts during and closes off the upper urethra. This means sperm are directed outwards at orgasm rather than passing back up into the bladder – a condition known as retrograde ejaculation.

BPH
What Is BPH?

From around the age of 45, the number of cells in the prostate gland increases and the gland starts to enlarge in most men. This is a non-cancerous process known as benign prostatic hyperplasia, or BPH for short. The word *hyperplasia* refers to an increase in the number of cells present in the prostate gland. As the number of cells increases, the prostate gland enlarges. The condition used to be known as benign prostatic hypertrophy, but this is no longer used as it is inaccurate – the word 'hypertrophy' implies that enlargement is due to an increase in the size of each cell rather an increase in the number of cells present, and this is not what actually occurs.

Research shows that BPH is mostly associated with an increase in the number of fibrous and muscle cells (known as *stroma*) that surround the millions of tiny gland cells within the prostate, rather than an increase in the number of gland (that is, secreting) cells. In a normal prostate, the ratio of fibre and muscle cells to gland cells is around 2:1. In BPH, this ratio increases to around 5:1. As the prostate enlarges, smooth muscle cells within the prostate also become slightly stretched. This triggers a reflex contraction so the general tone of the muscle cells increases.

BPH is a normal process and, in the early stages, is not classed as a disease. It is only when growth becomes greater than required and starts to affect urinary flow that symptoms start to arise. Symptoms usually start slowly, but once they are established can worsen quite quickly. Severe difficulties can arise within 10 years if steps are not taken to reduce enlargement of the prostate gland.

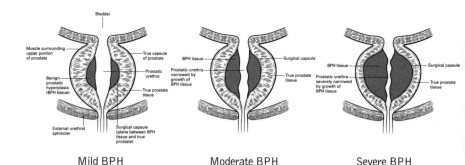

Mild BPH   Moderate BPH   Severe BPH

Symptoms

The urinary tube (urethra) leading from the bladder passes down through the centre of the prostate gland. In some men, the prostate gland grows large without causing problems with passing water. This may be because their urethra is wider than average, or because the gland tends to enlarge outwards rather than in. In many, however, enlargement of the prostate gland squeezes the urethra to interfere with urinary flow. Spasm of the stretched smooth muscle fibres within the gland also contribute to squeezing of the urethra and the development of a number of embarrassing urinary symptoms which doctors refer to as *prostatism*.

Symptoms of prostatism have two main causes:

1 narrowing of the prostatic urethra and muscular spasm of the prostate gland (obstructive symptoms)
2 irritation, stretching and thickening of the bladder as it tries to force urine past the blockage (irritative symptoms).

The Obstructive Symptoms of Prostatism

- straining or difficulty when starting to pass water (hesitancy)
- a weak urinary stream which may start and stop mid-flow
- dribbling of urine after voiding
- urinary retention

- having to rush to the toilet (urgency)
- passing water more often than normal (daytime frequency)
- having to get up to pass urine at night (nocturia)
- discomfort when passing water
- urinary incontinence
- a feeling of not having emptied the bladder fully

These irritative symptoms are often more troublesome than those due to narrowing of the urethra and interference with the urinary stream. The need to pass water at night disturbs the sleep of both the sufferer and his bed partner, which can lead to friction in a relationship – especially if sexual activity is also affected due to erectile dysfunction.

The size of the prostate gland does not necessarily relate to severity of symptoms, however. This depends on the direction in which the gland enlarges, and the width of the urinary tube that a man has inherited. In some, only a small enlargement in prostate size will squeeze the urethra enough to cause problems. In others, the gland may predominantly enlarge outwards so that even when it has reached a large size it does not significantly affect urinary flow.

PLEASE NOTE

Blood in the urine or sperm is *not* a usual symptom of BPH. If you notice this you must see your doctor as soon as possible, as this needs further investigation.

How Common Is It?

BPH is one of the most common medical conditions to affect men over the age of 50 years, and the single most common problem dealt with by urologists. One study[1] of over 700 men suggests that symptoms affect 14 per cent of men aged 40–49 years, and 50 per cent of men aged 60–69 years. Overall, it produced symptoms in 25 per cent of men aged 40–79 years. By the age of 80 it is estimated that as many as 80 per cent of men are affected. It has been estimated that a man aged 40 years has a 1 in 3 chance of undergoing a surgical operation for prostate enlargement during later life.

What Causes It?

Most researchers agree that enlargement of the prostate gland is linked with testosterone and its breakdown products. Testosterone is the sex hormone responsible for male characteristics. Ninety-five per cent of circulating testosterone is made in the testes from puberty onwards. The remaining 5 per cent is produced in the adrenal glands just above the kidneys.

Around 90 per cent of circulating testosterone is bound to protein (albumin and Sex Hormone Binding Globulin – SHBG) in the circulation, and it is only the unbound fraction that can enter prostate cells.

Once in the prostate cells, testosterone is converted into another, more powerful male hormone, dihydro-testosterone (DHT). This conversion is controlled by a prostate enzyme, 5-alpha-reductase. It is DHT that is responsible for triggering the division of prostate cells so their numbers increase. Levels of DHT are known to be 5 times higher in enlarged prostate glands than in those of normal size. If the conversion of testosterone to DHT is prevented, BPH does not occur and can even be reversed once it has developed.

There is a condition in which males lack the enzyme 5-alpha-reductase. As a result their genitals do not develop normally and initially remain so small they are often mistaken for girls until puberty. The penis and scrotum then suddenly enlarge and the voice deepens. A genetic deficiency of 5-alpha-reductase is relatively common in the Dominican Republic, where those affected are known as *guevedoces* – meaning 'penis at age 12'. Those affected only develop a tiny prostate gland, do not go bald and never suffer from acne – conditions which are also linked with testosterone and DHT.

TESTOSTERONE

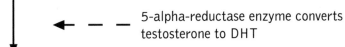 5-alpha-reductase enzyme converts testosterone to DHT

DIHYDRO-TESTOSTERONE (DHT)

PROSTATE GLAND GROWTH

The Effects of Testosterone Hormone

- stimulates male sex drive
- stimulates muscular development
- stimulates growth of the penis and testes
- stimulates sperm production
- stimulates growth of the male larynx so the voice deepens

The Effects of DHT

- stimulates growth of facial and body hair
- increases oil gland activity and encourages acne
- triggers male pattern baldness
- triggers benign enlargement of the prostate gland

Although the exact cause of prostate enlargement is unknown, it may be linked with the relative lowering of testosterone levels and the relative increase in oestrogen levels that occur with increasing age.[2] Certainly prostate size and volume are directly associated with oestrogen levels.[3] The prostate gland may respond to the changing hormone environment by enlarging to absorb more of the lower amount of testosterone available.

Some evidence also suggests that BPH may be an auto-immune problem, as antibodies aimed against prostate specific antigen (PSA – a prostate enzyme) appear to be much higher in men with BPH than in those with prostatitis and in men without prostate problems.[4]

An interesting new theory suggests that toxins produced by intestinal bacteria

(*E. coli*) which have found their way into the prostate gland may be the direct cause of the cell overgrowth that triggers BPH.[5] Certainly research in which prostate biopsies were examined under the microscope suggests that infection is present in a significant number of cases.[6] Of these, Gram-positive bacteria were found in 32.8 per cent of samples, gram-negative bacteria in 30.8 per cent and fungi in 2.9 per cent.

Recent studies have shown that inflammatory cells start to infiltrate the prostate gland as it enlarges, and as some of these cells produce chemicals that affect the growth and proliferation of other cells (growth factors) it is possible that these are also involved in the BPH process.

BPH and Baldness

Both BPH and male pattern baldness (androgenic alopecia) are linked with testosterone, 5-alpha-reductase and DHT. When 225 patients over 60 years old with BPH were compared with 160 similar men without BPH, the proportion of men with male pattern baldness (Grade IV or higher) was significantly greater in those with BPH than those without (53.8 per cent versus 36.9 per cent). There was also a greater frequency of men with inherited baldness among those with BPH.[7] This study was performed in North Korea, where both BPH and baldness are less common than in Western males.

BPH and Diet

BPH is more common in some races than in others. Men in China and Japan, for example, are at least 10 times less likely to develop BPH than men in the

Western world. This suggests that heredity plays a part, but diet is also thought to play an important role. One theory is that soya products and Oriental vegetables and grains in the diet help to protect those living in Eastern cultures from prostate enlargement. These dietary staples all contain weak, oestrogen-like hormones (known as phytoestrogens) which are released from food by the action of bacteria in the gut. These phytoestrogens are thought to affect the natural male hormone balance in the prostate gland to help protect against BPH. Blood levels of dietary oestrogens are significantly higher in Eastern men compared with those in the West. Soya protein found in Finnish bread seems to protect males in Finland too. Unfortunately, there are signs that Japanese and Chinese men who adopt a more Western diet, with increased intakes of total calories, fat and animal protein and decreased intakes of vegetables and wholegrains are losing their traditional protection against prostatic disease. For more information, see Chapter 4.

How BPH Can Affect Lifestyle

The symptoms of BPH can have a drastic effect on a man's life. Many men with prostate symptoms avoid drinking fluids at certain times. Some reduce their total fluid intake drastically, but this will only make symptoms worse. Dehydration makes urine stronger and more likely to cause irritation, infection, encourage bladder stone formation and increase unwanted odour. Many men also become depressed, develop low self-esteem and stop participating in social or leisure activities or travelling far afield due to the difficulty of having to find public toilets at short notice.

A study[8] of over 400 men aged 40–79 years with BPH found that 51 per cent reported that their symptoms interfered with at least one of a number of selected daily activities such as the amount of fluids they would take before travel or bedtime, sleep patterns, driving for more than two hours without a break, and venturing out to places without toilets, playing outdoor sports or visiting the cinema, theatre or church. For 17 per cent of these men, the interference occurred most or all of the time.

How BPH Can Affect Your Sex Life

A survey[9] of 800 men over the age of 50 years found that almost half of sexually active males with symptoms of prostatism experienced a lower sex drive, erectile dysfunction and problems with ejaculation. As a result, half as many men with prostate symptoms made love at least once a week compared with those without problems (20 per cent versus 40 per cent).

More recent research involving 168 men with BPH found that 59 per cent had a low sex drive, 56 per cent had infrequent erections (with 46 per cent fulfilling the criteria for impotence), while 38 per cent had ejaculation problems.

A study[10] of 423 men with BPH in the community and 1,271 men attending urology clinics also found that sexual problems were common. Rigidity of erections was reduced in 60 per cent of men with BPH (versus 53 per cent in the community), reduced ejaculation in 62 per cent (versus 47 per cent) and pain on ejaculation was experienced by 17 per cent (versus 5 per cent). Sex lives were admitted as spoiled by lower urinary tract symptoms in 8 per cent of men in the community and 46 per cent of those in the clinic.

There is obviously a high degree of sexual problems in men with prostate symptoms, and it is important that couples affected do not suffer in silence but seek help. Even if their doctor decides the symptoms of BPH do not warrant medical or surgical treatment, self-help with herbal remedies such as Saw Palmetto, Muira Puama, Catuaba and Ginkgo can help enormously. See Chapter 3. See also the book *Increase Your Sex Drive* by Dr Sarah Brewer (Thorsons).

What Happens If BPH Is Not Treated?

Because symptoms of prostatism tend to start slowly, many men assume they're a part of growing old and do not seek help. Surveys suggest that, on average, men suffering from prostatism wait four years before consulting their doctor about urinary problems. If a man suspects he has a prostate problem however, it is important to seek medical advice sooner rather than later. If left untreated, BPH can lead to infection (cystitis) due to stagnation of urine trapped in the bladder, the formation of bladder stones due to salts precipitating out of stagnant urine, a total inability to pass water (acute urinary retention) due to complete blocking of the urethra, and kidney damage due to back pressure and backflow of trapped urine.

BPH and Acute Retention of Urine

One of the most distressing complications of BPH is acute retention of urine. This occurs when the prostate enlarges enough to squeeze the urethra fully closed so that urine cannot pass out from the bladder. Acute retention of urine is often triggered by spasm of the bladder or pelvic muscles and is made worse by anxiety about not being able to pass water. As urine builds up in the bladder, stretch pains become unbearable and medical help is needed to help drain the urine – and bring instant relief. This is usually achieved by passing a catheter (flexible tube) into the bladder, through the penis, using a local anaesthetic gel to numb the sensitive urethra. Occasionally, if a catheter cannot be passed through the blockage and the urethra cannot be dilated using special rods, a suprapubic catheter has to be passed into the bladder through the overlying abdominal wall.

Increased awareness of the importance of seeking help for prostate problems means that this embarrassing, unpleasant and painful complication is now becoming less common.

What to Do If You Think You Have BPH

If you suspect you have symptoms of prostatism, it is important to tell your doctor as soon as possible. Don't wait until symptoms become troublesome and start interfering with your life. Early screening will help to prevent complications, and also means that the more serious, but potentially curable problem of prostate cancer is picked up early and treated sooner rather than later.

How to Assess the Severity of Symptoms

Two sets of guidelines have appeared over recent years to help doctors assess the severity of an individual's symptoms. In 1992, an International Consensus meeting drew up guidelines known as the International Prostate Symptoms Score (I-PSS) to grade the severity of prostate symptoms and their effect on quality of life.[11]

A man with prostate symptoms is asked to answer 6 questions as follows, marking off the appropriate answer to each one.

Over the past month, how often have you:	Not at all	<1 time in 5	<half the time	half the time	>half the time	almost always
1. Had a sensation of not emptying your bladder completely after you finished urination?	0	1	2	3	4	5
2. Had to urinate again less than two hours after you finished urinating?	0	1	2	3	4	5
3. Found you stopped and started again several times when you urinated?	0	1	2	3	4	5
4. Found it difficult to postpone urination?	0	1	2	3	4	5
5. Had a weak urinary stream?	0	1	2	3	4	5
6. Had to push or strain to begin urination?	0	1	2	3	4	5

He is then asked two additional questions:

Over the past month, how many times did you:	None	Once	Twice	3 times	4 times	5 or more times
Most typically get up to urinate from the time you went to bed at night until the time you got up in the morning?						

If you were to spend the rest of your life with your urinary condition just the way it is now:	Delighted	Pleased	Mostly satisfied	Mixed	Mostly dissatisfied	Terrible
How would you feel about that?						

The I-PSS combines the total score from these three questions to give an I-PSS value which can range from 0 to 41. A medical management plan based on the I-PSS and/or the findings of digital rectal examination (DRE – see pages 21–2), or blood test to measure the prostate specific antigen level (PSA – see page 24–6) is suggested as follows:

1 Watchful waiting is acceptable where the I-PSS value is less than 9.

2 Medical treatment of moderate BPH is suggested if:

the I-PSS is between 9 and 17

Prostate specific antigen (PSA) level is less than 4 ng/ml

Digital rectal examination (DRE) suggests benign enlargement

3 Referral is necessary if:

the I-PSS is greater than 17

the PSA is greater than 4 ng/ml

there is any suggestion of prostate malignancy on DRE.

The diagnostic criteria also suggests ruling out other conditions on the basis of medical history, a physical examination and blood tests to assess how well the kidneys are working.

'Watchful waiting' means that the patient does not receive any medial treatments, but is reviewed regularly to see if symptoms worsen. This is an ideal time to start taking Saw Palmetto extracts, as will be discussed further in Chapter 2.

The Shared-Care Initiative (SCI)

The Shared-Care Initiative[12] was suggested in 1993 by a UK working party which reviewed comments and ideas from around 2,000 doctors. This took the form of an algorithm designed to ensure that:

- patients with minimal symptoms of prostatism were not referred too early

- all men over 55 years are screened with 3 simple questions to identify those who may need treatment:
  - Are you bothered by urinary symptoms?
  - Is your urinary stream abnormal?
  - Do you have to pass water during the night?
- the 'worried well' or curious are taken seriously and assessed appropriately.

The Shared Care Initiative recognizes the fact that men worried about possible prostate problems need to be taken seriously, even if they do not currently have symptoms needing treatment. BPH is progressive, with symptoms that fluctuate over time and in some cases improve. The worried well must therefore be reassured that, although they may not need treatment at that time, they should return if symptoms worsen as they are likely to develop troublesome prostate symptoms in the future. If they do not feel that they will be taken seriously, they may become one of the many males whose prostate disease remains undiagnosed and untreated.

The SCI management flow chart, therefore, suggests that males who are curious about BPH as a result of media reports – or reading a book such as this – receive a base-line assessment including:

- full urological history to assess the severity of their symptoms
- physical and digital rectal examination
- urinalysis
- blood tests to assess kidney function.

Again, the so-called worried well are likely to benefit from taking a herbal supplement such as extracts of Saw Palmetto.

Medical Examination for BPH

When you tell your doctor you have a prostate problem, he or she will ask you detailed questions about your symptoms. It can help to have kept a urinary 'symptoms diary' for a week or so to record how often you experience urinary difficulties such as hesitancy, frequency and nocturia. The doctor will then examine you generally to assess your overall health, feel your abdomen to assess whether your kidneys or bladder are enlarged, then may briefly examine your genitals.

One of the most important parts of the physical examination is a digital rectal examination (DRE) to assess the size, shape and texture of your prostate gland. The doctor gently inserts a gloved and lubricated finger into your back passage – nowhere near as unpleasant an experience as many men fear. Most people describe the sensation as similar to slight constipation.

Usually the prostate feels smooth and firm, is 2–3 cm across and feels firm and rubbery. Usually two lobes can be felt, separated by an obvious groove running down the centre of the gland. In BPH, the prostate still feels smooth and firm but is obviously enlarged – sometimes to the size of a golf ball or even – exceptionally – to the size of a grapefruit. The anatomical groove may still be present.

DRE helps to confirm that the prostate is enlarged. It also helps to screen for prostatitis (in which the prostate may be 'boggy' and tender) and prostate cancer, which may be detected if the area in reach of the finger feels hard, craggy, irregular or is tethered to the overlying soft tissues. DRE cannot reliably differentiate between BPH and early prostate cancer, however. If a suspicious nodule is felt there is only a 50 per cent chance that a cancer is present, and unfortunately 36 per cent of patients dying from prostate cancer will not have a tumour that is detectable by routine DRE.

Investigations

Your doctor will usually request a few tests, which – depending on your symptoms and signs – may include:

- a full blood count to check for anaemia or infection
- kidney function tests (Urea and Electrolytes) to assess your salt balance
- measurement of prostate specific antigen (PSA) – which may be raised if there is a hidden prostate tumour (see page 24)
- prostatic acid phosphatase (PAP) – which may be raised in prostate cancer if secondaries have spread to the bones.

Urine Tests

Urine tests may be requested to check for sugar, protein, blood or signs of infection. They are not that helpful in BPH, however. They may detect blood (haematuria) where prostate cancer is present, and pus cells in prostatitis, but these are frequently normal in both conditions.

Measurement of Urinary Flow

Measurement of urinary flow rate helps to assess how badly your stream is affected. This involves passing urine into a bottle with a special by-pass, or into a funnel or toilet with an electronic device attached. The speed at which you pass urine and the total amount passed are printed out in the form of a graph (uroflowmetry). This will help to show how much your urinary outflow is obstructed, though around a quarter of men with urinary problems due to prostate enlargement will show no evidence of obstruction in pressure flow studies.

Your doctor might also refer you to a hospital specialist. This doesn't necessarily mean anything serious is wrong. It may simply be that your GP is unable to request some of the tests you need directly, or because local guidelines recommend review by a urologist.

Ultrasound

Ultrasound may be used to pass high-frequency, inaudible and painless sound waves through your body. These bounce back off tissue planes and are analysed by a computer to produce an image on a screen. Ultrasound can check the size of your prostate gland and kidneys and can also measure how much residual urine stays in your bladder after voiding. For a more direct assessment of the prostate gland, a lubricated, finger-shaped probe can be inserted gently into the back passage during transrectal ultrasound (TRUS). This test is especially helpful for assessing whether a nodule detected through DRE is solid or cystic, and to screen the prostate in males found to have a raised PSA (see page 24).

Transrectal Needle Biopsy

Transrectal needle biopsy (TRNB) may be suggested under ultrasound guidance, to allow biopsy of suspicious sites in the prostate gland so that cells can be obtained for examination under a microscope. The removal of fine cores of prostatic tissue is relatively painless with the new biopsy guns.

Cystoscopy

Cystoscopy (insertion of a narrow telescope into the bladder through the penis) may be recommended to view the urethra, bladder and the site of prostate obstruction in some cases. This procedure is also performed at the same time as surgical resection of the prostatic urethra to clear the blockage (see page 27).

Dye Tests

Dye tests in which the kidneys and urinary tract are outlined with substances that show up on x-ray (intravenous pyelogram – IVP – and excretory urograms) are now rarely needed due to advances in other techniques.

PSA Testing

Prostate specific antigen (PSA) is an enzyme, discovered in 1971, that is produced only by prostate cells and helps to liquefy semen by breaking down the clotted proteins produced by the seminal vesicles. PSA levels are undetectable in women and in men who have had their prostate gland removed.

A number of factors can raise the PSA level, including having BPH, certain drugs, and the presence of prostate cancer. It is a more sensitive indicator of prostate cancer than digital rectal examination (DRE) or transrectal ultrasound (TRUS). Only a quarter to one-third of asymptomatic males with a raised PSA will be found to have a prostate cancer, however.

If prostate cancer is suspected, a blood test is usually performed to measure circulating levels of the protein prostate specific antigen (PSA).

- If PSA is normal (0 to 4 ng/ml) there is only a 2.5 per cent chance that a man has prostate cancer.
- If it is moderately raised (between 4 and 10 ng/ml) there is a 20 per cent chance of prostate cancer.
- If the blood level is very raised (above 10 ng/ml) there is a greater than 50 per cent chance that cancer of the prostate is present.

Unfortunately, the interpretation of PSA levels is not straightforward. One in five men with prostate cancer have normal PSA levels, and 25 per cent of men without prostate cancer have raised levels. It does not diagnose whether or not a cancer is present, but gives an estimate of the risk that prostate cancer is present. It has been estimated that PSA testing plus DRE can increase the detection of cancer by 32 per cent over DRE alone.

Research is currently investigating whether a refinement of the test, which uses a correction factor known as PSA density, would be more specific. This refinement can only be used where the volume of the prostate has been assessed using TRUS, however. Using a series of PSA tests is likely to be more helpful than a single PSA measurement. When PSA levels rise by more than 20 per cent per year, for example, referral for prostate biopsy is recommended.

A newly discovered protein, known as protein D, has recently been identified in prostate fluid from men with prostate cancer, but not in those with normal prostate tissue or those with BPH.[13] This protein may prove a useful marker test for prostate cancer in the future.

Prostate Screening

There is currently much controversy over whether annual screening for prostate cancer is justified in the UK. This is because the PSA test is not highly specific nor highly sensitive for prostate cancer, so that false-positive and false-negative results can occur. Some researchers also feel that, because prostate cancer is often non-aggressive and is a disease many men will die with, rather than from, regular screening may lead to over-treatment, as there is currently little consensus on how to treat the early stages of the illness.

Studies have not clearly shown that early detection improves survival, but early detection may potentially lead to reduced morbidity and improved quality of life – especially in younger males. Attitudes are different in the US, where routine annual DRE is offered to all men aged 40 and over, plus yearly PSA tests beginning at the age of 50, or earlier (from age 40) for African Americans, who are at greater risk, and for those with a positive family history of prostate cancer.

Orthodox Treatment

Benign prostatic hyperplasia (BPH) is treated in three main ways, depending on the severity of symptoms and how much they interfere with quality of life: surgery, medication and herbal treatments.

Surgery

Surgery for BPH is known as transurethral resection of the prostate (TURP) and involves passing a narrow instrument (resectoscope) through the end of the penis under general anaesthetic. A fibre-optic light and lens system allow the surgeon to view the urethra directly and clear the blockage by paring away the bulging inner surface of the prostate gland. A high-frequency electric arc or a laser beam is used to trim away excess tissue and simultaneously cauterize bleeding points. A continuous, fluid irrigation system flushes the trimmings away and allows some to be collected for examination under a microscope. Histology reveals a hidden tumour in around 5 per cent of cases.

After surgery it usually takes several weeks for symptoms to settle down. Up to 20 per cent of men will have post-operative problems with intermittent, dribbling incontinence of urine. In about 5 per cent of cases this problem is continuous. The prostate usually continues to enlarge so symptoms recur and 15 per cent of men require further surgery within eight years of the first operation.

There is no obvious reason why surgery for TURP should affect a man's sex drive or ability to maintain an erection. A few men do seem to experience sexual problems after the operation, however, and around half notice a change in the intensity of orgasm. Between 30 and 90 per cent of men also develop retrograde ejaculation after prostate surgery, so that sperm pass backwards into the bladder during ejaculation. This is not harmful and sperm are passed along with urine next time the bladder is emptied. The condition does cause infertility however, and medical assistance is needed if the affected male wishes to father a child.

Other surgical measures include inserting a tubular metal mesh into the prostatic urethra, balloon dilation of the prostatic urethra, or using microwaves, ultrasound or hot needles to heat shrink the gland.

Occasionally an open operation is performed for BPH, in which the entire prostate gland is shelled out through an incision over the pubic bone. This may be needed when the prostate is very enlarged, there are large bladder stones that need removal, or where a potentially curable prostate cancer is also present. The risk of erectile dysfunction and retrograde ejaculation are greater with open prostatectomy than with TURP.

Quality of life for patients with prostatism only improves for those with severe symptoms. As most surgery is carried out on men with mild to moderate symptoms of BPH, it has been said that the majority will unfortunately not notice a great impact on their lives.[14]

Using Medication to Shrink the Gland

The drug finasteride is designed to shrink the prostate gland by blocking 5-alpha-reductase, the enzyme needed to convert the male hormone, testosterone, to dihydro-testosterone. This can help an enlarged prostate gland to shrink by over 20 per cent and is particularly beneficial to men with severe symptoms. It takes time to work, however, and treatment usually needs to be taken continuously as the prostate may start to grow within a few weeks of stopping the tablets.

As the drug has a hormonal action, it is important to use condoms to protect any sexual partners from exposure to the drug in the man's semen.

Using Medication to Relax the Gland

A number of drugs are designed to relax the smooth muscle cells in the prostate gland so that constriction due to spasm is relieved. The first drugs used to do this – known as selective alpha-blockers (such as prazosin, terazosin, indoramin) – were originally developed to treat high blood pressure. They work by damping down nervous system activity which triggers contraction of muscle fibres in the prostate and urethra. By relaxing these muscles, the urethral bore is widened to improve symptoms.

A newer class of drug, the $\alpha 1A$-adrenoceptor antagonists (such as tamsulosin) has recently been developed specifically to treat BPH and is less likely to cause problems such as dizziness due to low blood pressure. These $\alpha 1A$-adrenoceptor antagonists work by targeting a specific receptor in the prostate tissue (the $\alpha 1A$-adrenoceptor) to encourage the gland to relax.

Using Medication to Relax the Bladder

If symptoms are mainly irritative rather than obstructive, drugs that reduce irritation and spasm of the bladder (such as oxybutynin, flavoxate, propantheline) can help to relieve symptoms such as frequency of passing urine, urgency and incontinence. They should not be used if the prostate is greatly enlarged, however, so are of limited value in treating BPH.

Natural Herbal Treatments

A variety of natural herbal treatments are available for helping symptoms of BPH. Of these, Saw Palmetto berry extracts are the most widely researched (see Chapters 2 and 3). It is important to always tell your doctor if you develop urinary symptoms, as BPH needs to be diagnosed and prostate cancer ruled out before you decide whether or not to take a herbal supplement such as Saw Palmetto.

Prostatitis

The millions of tiny glands present in the prostate secrete fluids into a wide-spread system of passageways that can become clogged, infected or inflamed to produce prostatitis.

Clogging may be due to the production of thicker secretions than normal, or the formation of tiny, gravel-like stones. In one case,[15] an 83-year-old man with prostatitis was found to have 125 stones in his prostate gland weighing a total of 28 g! Prostatitis is more often due to infection, however, which may be due to bowel or skin bacteria that find their way into the gland, or to sexually transmissible diseases such as Chlamydia, gonorrhoea or Ureaplasma. Inflammation can also occur as a result of chemical irritation if urine refluxes up into its passageways. This is thought to be most likely as a result of jogging or exercising with a full bladder, which should be avoided.

There are three main types of prostatitis:

1 acute (recent onset) bacterial infection

2 chronic (long-term) bacterial infection

3 chronic (long-term) non-bacterial inflammation.

An estimated one in three men suffers from prostatitis at some time between the ages of 20 and 50 years. Some research, in which prostate biopsies were examined under the microscope, suggests that prostatitis is present in as many as 90 per cent of men with BPH.[16] Of these, Gram-positive bacteria were found in 32.8 per cent of samples, gram-negative bacteria in 30.8 per cent, and fungi in 2.9 per cent. In 27.9 per cent of samples no infective organisms could be obtained, although there was real evidence of prostatitis.

Symptoms vary and may include:

- feeling unwell, sometimes with chills or fever
- aching round the thighs, genitals or lower back
- deep pain between the scrotum and anus
- pain and difficulty on passing water
- passing water more frequently
- pain on ejaculation
- discharge from the penis which may be watery or stained with blood or pus
- sometimes nausea and vomiting.

Unfortunately, chronic prostatitis – which affects around one in 100 men – can be difficult to treat and some men suffer recurrent symptoms throughout their life.

When suffering from prostatitis, either avoid sex or use condoms in case infection is present. Your doctor will advise on when you can resume normal sexual relations.

How Prostatitis Is Investigated

Prostatitis is best investigated by doctors specializing in urology or genito-urinary medicine, as a complete screen for urinary tract infections — including sexually transmissible diseases — is needed. Digital rectal examination may reveal a tender prostate gland that feels soft, but often findings are normal. Swabs collect penile discharge for examination under the microscope, and for laboratory culture, including special immune tests to detect Chlamydia infection.

A special three-glass test is sometimes performed for suspected prostatitis. You will be asked to pass a small amount of urine into one glass jar, and more into a second jar. These samples are checked for cloudiness, blood and for threads of cellular material that suggests urethral inflammation. After passing urine into the second jar, you are asked to stop voiding and retain some urine. The doctor then inserts a gloved finger into your rectum and gently massages the prostate gland to release any secretions trapped inside. You will then be asked to pass a small sample of urine into a third glass jar, to flush through the released prostate fluids.

The three-glass test aims to distinguish between infection in different parts of the male urogenital tract. The results are not always clear-cut, but in general:

- If bacteria are found in the first glass jar, this suggests infection of the urethra (the tube leading from the bladder to the opening at the tip of the penis).

- If bacteria are present in the second sample, this suggests a possible bladder infection (cystitis).

- If more bacteria are found in the third glass jar than in the first, this suggests prostatitis.
- If pus cells but no significant bacteria are present in the third glass jar, this suggests non-bacterial prostatitis.

Treatment of Prostatitis

Once an infection is suspected or diagnosed, a prolonged course of antibiotic tablets are prescribed, usually for at least 4 weeks. Symptoms should start to improve within a few days.

Chronic infection can be difficult to treat, as inflammation and swelling traps infection inside the gland. Antibiotics are often prescribed for at least six weeks and sometimes for three months or longer. Non-steroidal anti-inflammatory painkillers such as ibuprofen can help to damp down swelling, inflammation and pain.

Chronic prostatitis often responds well to natural herbal remedies such as Rye grass extracts and evening primrose oil. See Chapter 3.

Prostatodynia

Prostatodynia literally means 'prostate pain'. The condition – which is some-times also known as vegetative-urogenital-syndrome – causes unpleasant symptoms of recurrent discomfort in the lower abdomen, scrotum, testicles, groin, penis and in the region of the prostate gland. There is no evidence of inflammation or infection.

The exact cause is unknown, but it is widely thought that spasm of the pelvic floor muscles accounts for the fact that urinary flow is often abnormally slow and starting urination is difficult. It may also be associated with sexual problems such as pain on erection or ejaculation, or impotence. Symptoms are often worse when ejaculation is infrequent, which suggests pain may be due to engorgement of the prostate gland, perhaps with secretions that are thicker than normal. It also seems to be triggered in some men by anxiety. Another possibility is that prostatodynia is due to irritation or malfunction of the nerves supplying the prostate gland.

Relief is often obtained by relaxation exercises, and from sitting in a hot bath for half an hour. Regular exercise and a high-fibre diet to keep the bowels regular are important for men with prostatodynia, as prolonged sitting and constipation increase prostate congestion. Try to avoid smoking, as this can trigger muscle spasm which may make symptoms worse. Some men find symptoms are aggravated by alcohol or caffeine.

Natural herbal remedies such as rye pollen extracts can help (see Chapter 3).

Prostate Cancer

Prostate cancer will affect 1 in 12 British men, 1 in 11 American white men and 1 in 10 American black men, who have the highest rate of this disease in the world.

Prostate cancer develops when a single cell within the gland escapes from the mechanisms controlling its normal growth and development. It then divides uncontrollably, rather than occasionally to replace old, worn-out prostate cells or in response to hormone triggers. In some cases the immune system recognizes and destroys these abnormal cells. If unchecked, however, the abnormal cells continue to divide and may eventually produce a detectable prostate cancer.

The growth of prostate cancer cells is now known to be linked with the action of male hormones (androgens), female hormones (oestrogens), glucocorticoid hormones and a variety of different growth factors, some of which are similar to insulin and which directly stimulate abnormal cell division under the influence of sex hormones.

Plant hormones such as genistein, found in soya beans, and some similar to that found in Saw Palmetto (beta-sitosterol) are thought to protect against prostate cancer because they interfere with this stimulatory action by influencing both the hormone and growth factor signaling pathways[17] (see Chapter 4).

Because there is increased cell activity in a prostate gland that is expanding due to benign prostatic hyperplasia (BPH), prostate cancer seems to be more likely in a prostate gland that is affected by BPH than one of normal size. Prostate cancer tends to arise in the same part of the prostate as BPH, and a condition known as atypical adenomatous hyperplasia is thought to be a possible intermediate stage between a BPH cell becoming a prostate cancer cell.[18] Most prostate cancers (83.3 per cent) arise in glands also affected by BPH, and around 10 per cent of men with BPH will be found to have prostate cancer on surgical treatment of their BPH.[19] For every male who develops prostate cancer, however, five more will suffer from benign enlargement (hyperplasia) of the gland and not develop prostate cancer.

Even when prostate cancer develops, it is not necessarily a death sentence. It features on the list of the 10 most survivable male cancers, and 43 per cent of men are still alive five years after the condition was first diagnosed.

Prostate cancer does seem to run in families, although less than 5 per cent of men with prostate cancer have a family history of the problem. One study[20] found that men with a first-degree relative (father or brother) affected are twice as likely to develop prostate cancer as men with no relatives affected. If a second-degree relative (uncle, grandfather) had prostate cancer as well, a man's risk increases to eight times that of a male with no affected relatives. Men with either two or three first-degree relatives affected have a 5-fold and 11-fold increased risk of developing prostate cancer respectively.

Prostate cancer is now among the most common male cancers in the West, and its incidence is increasing annually around the world by 2 to 3 per cent. It features in the list of the top two to four male cancers in most Western countries, where it is estimated that a man's lifetime risk of developing prostate cancer is around one in 11.

In the East, however, the incidence of prostate cancer is much lower: 26-fold lower in China and 10-fold lower in Japan.[21]

Relative National Differences in Prostate Cancer Frequency per 100,000 Males

China	1.8
Senegal	4.3
Singapore	4.8
Japan	6.7
India	8.2
England and Wales	18.1
Italy	18.8

Scotland	26.5
Finland	34.2
Sweden	45.9
Switzerland	50.1
US (white males)	53.4
US (black males)	91.2

There is more than a 50-fold difference between the rate of prostate cancer in China and that for black American males.

Interestingly, examination of prostate tissue at autopsy shows that the number of cases of prostate cancer is similar in both Asian and Western males, with prostate cancer cells found in 10 to 30 per cent of men aged 50–60 years and 50 to 70 per cent of men aged 70–80 years. For some reason, however, prostate cancers are more likely to remain small, slow-growing, clinically insignificant and undiagnosed in Eastern males. While this could be related to genetic influences this seems unlikely, as when native Japanese men migrate to the West their risk of clinically significant prostate cancer quickly rises so that within two generations it is the same as that of Western males.[22] This suggests that environmental factors are involved, and the most likely culprit is thought to be diet (see Chapter 4).

Unfortunately, the majority of prostate cancers arise in the outer parts of the prostate gland and tend not to obstruct urinary flow unless the tumour reaches a considerable size. It is therefore difficult to diagnose in the early stages. If obstructive symptoms do occur, they are similar to those of BPH but tend to progress more rapidly, over weeks rather than months. Nocturia and blood in the urine (haematuria) are also more likely. In the later stages of the disease, non-specific symptoms of cancer may occur, such as tiredness, weight loss, anaemia, swollen glands or pain.

Men who want to reduce their risk of prostate cancer, and those who have already been diagnosed with the disease, are likely to benefit by following the dietary advice given in Chapter 4.

Saw Palmetto

Saw Palmetto is a popular and effective traditional herbal remedy for male urinary discomfort caused by an enlarged prostate gland. It has long been hailed as
a male tonic, sexual rejuvenator and aphrodisiac, and is the most widely studied
natural herbal remedy for treating symptoms caused by benign prostatic hyperplasia (BPH). It has been used by Native Americans in Florida, where the tree
was originally found, to treat erectile problems, underactive testicles, symptoms
caused by benign prostatic hyperplasia (BPH) and inflammation (prostatitis)
for several hundred years. While it is likely to be helpful for many men with urinary problems, it is important that they always seek medical advice for a proper
diagnosis before self-treating.

The Plant

Saw Palmetto is an attractive, small palm tree that is native to the West Indies
and the Atlantic coast of North America, especially Florida, Georgia, Louisiana
and South Carolina. It grows from 1.8 to 3.3 metres (6 to 10 feet) high and is
popularly known as the dwarf American palm tree. Botanically, it has two
names: *Sabal serrulata* and *Serenoa repens,* and is also sometimes referred to as
Serenoa serrulata or *Sabalis serrulatae.* Not surprisingly, this has led to some

confusion among users and herbalists alike. In some cases, men have taken both a *Sabal serrulata* supplement and one containing *Serenoa repens*. Although this is unlikely to be harmful, it is unnecessarily expensive.

The tree is a member of the fan palm family and forms multiple fans of yellow-green, spiny-toothed leaves that are 60 cm (2 feet) long or more. It has ivory flowers that develop a dark berry fruit with a nutty, vanilla flavour. It is only the Saw Palmetto berry that is active against BPH, and it is important to choose a supplement that is licensed, or which contains a standardized amount of the berry extracts.

Unfortunately, the price of these raw extracts has increased significantly in recent years as demand has increased. Don't be tempted by the many cheaper supplements available, as these often do not contain enough of the active ingredients. Some which are labelled as containing Saw Palmetto extracts (rather than Saw Palmetto berry or fruit extracts) may, in fact, only contain powdered leaves and stalks, which will have no beneficial effect on the urinary system at all.

The active components of the Saw Palmetto fruits are found in the fat-soluble extracts. These contain a variety of essential fatty acids (EFAs), hormone-like substances (sterols such as β-sitosterol, campesterol and stigmasterol), polyphenic compounds and flavonoids. These extracts (often described as liposterolic extracts) are so effective at improving urinary flow and encouraging better bladder voiding in men with benign prostatic hyperplasia (BPH) that the Saw Palmetto is often referred to as the male *plant catheter*. The berry extracts can:

- reduce outflow obstruction in BPH
- strengthen the bladder neck
- produce a diuretic action
- improve urinary flow
- relieve urinary discomfort
- control urinary frequency.

What Saw Palmetto Can Do

Over 20 randomized, double-blind, placebo-controlled trials have shown that standardized extracts of Saw Palmetto berries providing 85 to 90 per cent fatty acids and sterols are effective in relieving the symptoms of BPH, especially night-time urinary frequency (nocturia). Double-blind, placebo-controlled studies involve one group of volunteers receiving the active ingredient, while another similar group receives an inactive look-alike substance known as placebo. Neither the volunteers nor the doctors are aware who is getting which treatment until the code is broken and the results analysed at the end of the trial. These results are therefore unbiased, and show whether or not the active ingredient is really better than placebo, rather than its effects being due to wishful thinking.

To summarize these findings, extracts of *Serenoa repens* have been found to:

- reduce urinary frequency at night (nocturia) by 33 to 74 per cent (versus 13 to 39 per cent with placebo)
- reduce urinary frequency during the day by 11 to 43 per cent (versus 1 to 29 per cent with placebo)

- increase peak urinary flow rate by 26 to 50 per cent (versus 2 to 35 per cent with placebo)
- reduce the amount of residual urine in the bladder after voiding by 50 per cent compared with a 9 per cent worsening in those on placebo.

Overall, both physicians and patients rated the effectiveness of treatment as good or very good in over 80 per cent of cases. Good to excellent tolerability was reported by more than 95 per cent of volunteers. Mild gastrointestinal side-effects such as nausea and abdominal pain were reported in less than 2 per cent of patients, and no serious side-effects have occurred.

Some of the more recent trials are detailed at the end of this chapter for those who are interested, although it does make rather dry reading!

Meta-analysis

One of the best ways of evaluating the mixed results of a number of studies is a meta-analysis, which pools data from comparable trials to give an average of the results from as many patients as possible. This method was applied to studies involving Saw Palmetto in 1998[1] and the results published in the prestigious *Journal of the American Medical Association*. A total of 18 studies involving 2,939 men were found to meet the inclusion criteria, in which:

- participants had to have symptoms of BPH
- treatment involved Saw Palmetto alone or in combination with other phytotherapeutic (herbal) substances

- a control group received inactive placebo or a comparison drug therapy for BPH
- treatment was given for at least 30 days.

The average length of treatment was 9 weeks (ranging in the 18 studies from 4–48 weeks). Compared with men receiving inactive placebo, Saw Palmetto extracts improved urinary tract symptoms by 28 per cent, nocturia by 25 per cent, peak urine flow by 24 per cent, mean urine flow by 28 per cent and residual urine volume by 43 per cent.

Men taking Saw Palmetto extracts were also more than twice as likely to report improvement in symptoms than men taking placebo. In the trials where Saw Palmetto was compared with the drug finasteride, men in both groups showed similar improvements in urinary symptoms and flow measures, but there was a significantly lower rate of erectile dysfunction. Of the men taking finasteride, 4.9 per cent experienced difficulties with erections, compared with only 1.1 per cent of those taking Saw Palmetto. Other unwanted side-effects were also mild and infrequent with Saw Palmetto. Overall, 7 per cent of men taking placebo, 9 per cent of those taking Saw Palmetto and 11 per cent of those taking the drug finasteride withdrew from the trials.

The researchers analysed all the data and concluded that there was evidence that Saw Palmetto improves urological symptoms and flow rates, and that, compared with finasteride, Saw Palmetto produces similar improvements in urinary tract symptoms but is associated with fewer adverse side-effects. Further research is needed, however, to determine Saw Palmetto's long-term effectiveness and whether or not it can prevent some of the complications associated with BPH.

A German urologist has also reviewed the effectiveness of three synthetic prescribed drugs with Saw Palmetto fruit extracts, based on various published studies.[2] He showed that the increase in peak urinary flow rate in long-term studies was around three times more impressive with Saw Palmetto extracts than with the synthetic drugs, as follows:

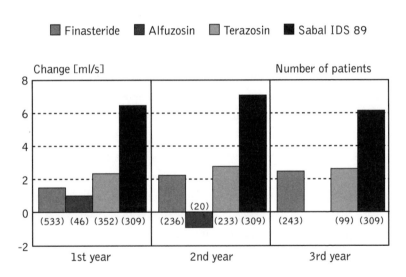

Increase in peak urinary flow rate in long-term studies with finasteride. From: Bach, D. *et al.* Phytropharmaceutical and Synthetic Agents in the Treatment of BPH.

In yet another medical review,[3] it was concluded that '... available data indicate that Serenoa repens is a useful alternative to alpha-one receptor antagonists (i.e. alpha-blockers) and finasteride in the treatment of men with BPH.'

How Saw Palmetto Works

The exact way in which Saw Palmetto works is unknown, although there are lots of theories. While Saw Palmetto does not alter the level of testosterone hormone circulating in the blood,[4] extracts from the fruit do significantly affect testosterone metabolism in cells taken from prostates affected by either BPH or prostate cancer.[5]

Does Saw Palmetto Block the Action of 5-alpha-reductase Enzyme?

Although it has been suggested that Saw Palmetto may block the action of the prostate enzyme 5-alpha-reductase, which converts the male hormone testosterone to the more powerful hormone dihydro-testosterone (DHT), this is controversial. A trial[6] that measured blood levels of DHT found no reduction in levels after eight days, but this does not rule out the possibility of local inhibitory effects in the prostate gland itself – or the possibility that effects take longer than eight days to develop.

Two studies have found Saw Palmetto to be a powerful inhibitor of 5-alpha-reductase in the laboratory, reducing the enzyme's activity by as much as 45 per cent.[7,8] This action has also been shown in cancerous prostate cells in the laboratory.[9] In a later study, therapeutic doses of Saw Palmetto extracts were found to inhibit the 5-alpha-reductase enzyme three times more strongly than the prescription-only drug finasteride.[10] Significant reductions in the production of DHT and increases in prostate testosterone levels were also found in biopsies from men who had taken *Serenoa repens* extracts for three months.[11] The researchers stated in their conclusions that the decrease of DHT and the rise of testosterone found in BPH tissue samples from men treated with *Serenoa repens* confirmed its ability to inhibit 5-alpha-reductase. These effects were especially noticeable in the tissues directly surrounding the urinary tube (peri-urethral tissue). It is therefore possible that *Serenoa* acts mainly on this central portion of the prostate, and only shrinks this area, which would explain why studies do not show appreciable shrinking of the whole gland despite significant improvements in urinary flow and obstructive symptoms.

Interestingly, two different types of 5-alpha-reductase enzyme are known to exist in the human prostate: isoenzymes type 1 and 2, with the type 2 enzyme predominating. It seems that the 5-alpha-reductase-blocking drug, finasteride, mainly inhibits the type 2 enzyme, while Saw Palmetto fruit extracts have been shown to inhibit both of the enzymes.[12]

Some believe it is more likely that Saw Palmetto extracts compete with DHT hormone for 'landing sites' on certain receptors so that, overall, prostate cells detect less DHT in the gland, even if levels of DHT are not greatly reduced. This competitive binding of Saw Palmetto extracts has been shown in fibre-producing cells (fibroblasts) extracted from human donated foreskins in the laboratory,[13] and in rat prostate cells.[14]

The controversy about whether or not Saw Palmetto extracts can interfere with the action of the 5-alpha-reductase enzymes continues, but a mounting body of evidence suggests that at least part of its effectiveness is due to this action.

Saw Palmetto Blocks the Effects of Oestrogen

As well as affecting the metabolism of testosterone in the prostate gland, Saw Palmetto also seems to reduce the effects of oestrogen.

One of the most interesting studies into the way Saw Palmetto works involved 35 men with BPH who were due to have an operation to remove their prostate gland. Three months before surgery, 18 patients were randomized to receive either Saw Palmetto fruit extracts or inactive placebo. Altogether, 18 men took *Serenoa repens* (160 mg three times a day) for three months up until the day before operation, and 17 took identical-looking inactive tablets. Neither the patients nor doctors knew who was taking what (that is, the trial was double-blind). After removal, the 35 prostate glands were examined in the laboratory and the number and type of hormone receptors in the prostate cells was analysed. In the men who did not take active treatment, oestrogen receptors were found in the nucleus of the prostate cells in 14 out of 17 cases, and in the main body of the prostate cells in 12 out of 17 cases. In the men who had taken the active Saw Palmetto extract, however, oestrogen receptors could not be detected in the nucleus of the cells in 17 out of the 18 men, and could only be detected in the main body of the cells in 6 out of the 18 cases. A significant reduction in progesterone hormone receptors was also found.

Hormone receptors are needed for hormones to produce an effect within cells, and by reducing the number of oestrogen and progesterone receptors present, the hormonal environment of the prostate gland becomes very different. It seems that Saw Palmetto extracts produce a significant anti-oestrogen effect[15] within the prostate gland, and this is probably important in reducing swelling.

Saw Palmetto Is an Alpha-Blocker

Some of the most effective prescription drugs used to treat BPH symptoms are known as alpha-blockers because they interact with a type of nerve-ending known as an alpha-receptor. This interaction triggers the relaxation of smooth muscle cells which, in the prostate, reduces spasm and improves urinary symptoms by widening the urinary outlet. Researchers have now discovered that Saw Palmetto berry extracts also have alpha-blocker abilities which is at a level only slightly lower than that of some prescribed alpha-blocker drugs.[16] This newly discovered activity undoubtedly contributes towards the effectiveness of Saw Palmetto.

Other Possible Actions

Several other of Saw Palmetto's actions have also been discovered, although the relative importance of each is not fully understood. These include the alteration of cholesterol metabolism[17] and the inhibition of another prostate enzyme, 3-ketosteroid reductase, which blocks the binding of dihydro-testosterone to prostate cells. Relaxation of the smooth muscle cells found in the bladder neck and in the prostate gland itself is also thought to account for some of the improvement in symptoms. Saw Palmetto is able to do this through a number of complex intracellular effects. The most important of these seems to be its action in blocking the movement of calcium ions in and out of the cells, as the movement of calcium is vital for muscle cells to contract.[18]

Some research also shows that Saw Palmetto fruit extracts have an anti-inflammatory action similar to that of aspirin and ibuprofen, by inhibiting an enzyme (cyclo-oxygenase) that is needed to make inflammatory chemicals.[19] This suggests that Saw Palmetto may be effective in treating prostatitis, although there has been little clinical work to investigate this.

There is no doubt that Saw Palmetto extracts are as effective as some pre-scription drugs in reducing the symptoms of BPH by encouraging an enlarged prostate gland to relax and shrink. The exact way in which it works is still poorly understood, but however it works, it does seem to reduce proliferation of prostate cells to improve symptoms of BPH – and this interference with the growth of prostate cells has even been shown to occur when cells have been stimulated to grow by a powerful growth factor.[20]

Prevention

Saw Palmetto is widely used to prevent prostate problems as well as to treat them. Many products containing extracts carry a statement along the lines of 'Helps to maintain a healthy prostate gland'. Certainly it ought to be effective in preventing prostate enlargement, as it definitely interferes with the metabolism of testosterone within prostate cells,[21] and has also been shown to neutralize the effects of growth factors on prostate cells. Unfortunately there have been no long-term trials to assess this action, and its use in preventing BPH is currently based on anecdotal evidence and faith alone. Given that 80 per cent of men will eventually develop symptoms caused by BPH, a preventive treatment is desperately needed. Studies are likely to be funded in the near future, but results would not be expected for many decades to come.

As Saw Palmetto is effective in treating symptoms once they start, there is an argument in favour of forgetting about prevention and just starting to take it as soon as mild urinary symptoms appear – after having had a medical check-up to confirm that it is BPH that is causing the problem. Many men in their early 40s are starting to take combined vitamin, mineral and Saw Palmetto supplements as part of their general health and fitness regime. This is unlikely to do any harm, and may well do a lot of good.

Dose

It is important to select only a reputable product containing standardized extracts of Saw Palmetto berry, as it is only these that will contain the active, fat-soluble sterols.

Cheaper products that may just be labelled 'Saw Palmetto extracts' may just contain powdered leaves and stalks, and will be no better than placebo. Similarly, alcoholic tinctures of Saw Palmetto do not provide significant levels of active compounds.

Fruit extracts	150 mg to 3 g daily in divided doses
Extracts providing 5:1 concentration (95 mg equivalent to 475 mg)	2 tablets three times a day.
Products standardized for 85 to 95 per cent fat-soluble sterols	320 mg daily.

A beneficial effect usually starts within two to six weeks, although some men notice an improvement almost straight away. Saw Palmetto extracts may be taken for as long as improvement is being achieved.

No significant side-effects have been reported.

Saw Palmetto in Combination with Other Natural Treatments

An increasing number of products are combining Saw Palmetto berry extracts with other natural ingredients for a potentially greater benefit. Saw Palmetto berry and nettle root, for example, are frequently combined (giving 320 mg of Saw Palmetto and 240 mg of nettle root per day).

Saw Palmetto has also been combined with evening primrose oil and the plant-derived hormone beta-sitosterol – the active ingredient in most plant-based prostate remedies – for additional anti-5-alpha-reductase activity.

The prosexual herbs Muira Puama and Damiana are also said to work synergistically with Saw Palmetto as prosexual supplements in men who have sexual problems such as low sex drive and erectile dysfunction (impotence) associated with prostate problems.

For more information about other herbs used to treat prostate problems, see Chapter 3.

PLEASE NOTE

Never diagnose prostate problems yourself – always seek medical advice if you develop urinary symptoms. If your doctor recommends a 'wait and see' approach you can start a prostate-friendly programme which includes taking

Saw Palmetto. If your doctor recommends taking a drug, remember you can choose to try a natural herbal extract first, instead, which has been shown to be just as effective as prescribed drugs but without the side-effects. You may even choose to take both the drug and herbal remedy together – but do let your doctor know if you intend to do this.

Results of Various Trials into the Effectiveness of Saw Palmetto Fruit Extracts

Unfortunately, this section of the chapter makes rather dry reading, but does help to underline the extent of the evidence that makes Saw Palmetto berry extracts the most widely prescribed treatment for BPH by doctors in many parts of Continental Europe.

In a double-blind trial involving 110 men with prostate symptoms, having to pass water at night (nocturia) decreased by an average of more than 45 per cent, flow rate increased by over 50 per cent and the amount of urine left in the bladder after voiding decreased by 42 per cent in those taking Saw Palmetto for 30 days. In contrast, those taking inactive placebo experienced only a 15 per cent reduction in nocturia, a 5 per cent increase in flow rate and a 9 per cent worsening of residual urinary volume.[22] Of those receiving Saw Palmetto extracts, their doctors rated their condition as greatly improved in 14 out of 50 cases, improved in 31 out of 50 cases and unchanged or worsened in only 5 out of 50 cases. In comparison, none of the men taking placebo were rated as greatly improved.

A placebo-controlled study[23] of 176 patients showed significant improvement in both day and night-time urinary frequency plus a significant increase in urinary flow rate after taking Saw Palmetto extracts for 60 days.

In a large uncontrolled study of over 1,330 patients in Germany, where these patients received 160 mg Saw Palmetto extracts twice a day for six months, the amount of urine remaining in the bladder after voiding was reduced by 50 per cent, frequency was reduced by 37 per cent, and nocturia by 54 per cent. Overall, both physicians and patients rated the effectiveness of treatment as good or very good in over 80 per cent of the cases.[24] Good to excellent tolerability was reported by more than 95 per cent of volunteers.

A trial[25] involving 46 men with previously untreated urinary symptoms caused by BPH and an International Prostate Symptoms Score (IPSS – see page 000) of 10 or more were given Saw Palmetto extracts of 160 mg twice a day for six months. The average IPSS improved from 19.5 to 12.5 over two months, and by more than 50 per cent for almost half of patients (46 per cent) by the end of the study. The researchers did not find any significant changes in urinary flow rate, but concluded that more placebo-controlled trials were warranted to evaluate the true effectiveness of Saw Palmetto.

A study[26] of 38 men with BPH showed that, after 12 months' treatment with Saw Palmetto fruit extracts, urinary symptoms improved in almost 75 per cent of cases. Average peak flow rates increased from 10.36 ml/s to 14.44 ml/s, and urinary retention after voiding decreased or disappeared in over 90 per cent of cases. Interestingly, the average volume of the prostate reduced by 10.6 per cent, which suggests a significant shrinking of prostate's size. This is unusual, however, as symptoms usually improve with Saw Palmetto berry extracts without appreciable changes in prostate volume.

A three-year trial[27] showed that peak urinary flow rate increased by an average of 6.1 ml/s and residual urinary volume left in the bladder after passing water decreased by 50 per cent. Improvement in quality of life was rated as good or very good in over 80 per cent of cases. Unfortunately, this study was not placebo-controlled, which reduces its value as critics could argue that many of the benefits were caused by the placebo effect.

In a study[28] of 339 men with BPH who took Saw Palmetto for three months, only 5.9 per cent of the men were delighted, happy or satisfied with their quality of life at the start of the trial. By Day 45 of the study, 43 per cent were delighted, happy or satisfied, rising to 76.3 per cent of men by Day 90. Interestingly, blood levels of PSA (see page 24) decreased significantly between Day 1 and Day 90. Overall, 80 per cent of patients judged the effects of Saw Palmetto fruit extracts as good or excellent.

How Saw Palmetto Compares with Prescription Drugs

A few studies have compared Saw Palmetto extracts with prescription drugs to see how effective they are in relation to one another.

In a randomized, controlled trial[29] of over 1,000 patients which compared extracts of Saw Palmetto with a prescription-only drug, finasteride, both treatments achieved a 38 per cent decrease in BPH symptoms over a six-month period. Interestingly, however, sexual function in the men using the natural treatment did not change, although it deteriorated significantly in those taking the prescribed medication. Saw Palmetto extracts, therefore, seem to be as effective as the prescribed drug for relieving symptoms of BPH, but without the undesirable side-effects of low sex drive and impotence.

In a study[30] that compared the action of Saw Palmetto extracts with a prescribed alpha-blocker drug, prazosin, 25 patients took the drug while 20 patients took *Serenoa repens* extracts for 12 weeks. The flow rate and symptoms improved in both groups to a similar extent, although the improvements in irritative symptoms (see page 8) were slightly less with Saw Palmetto.

A study[31] of 63 men with BPH who received either Saw Palmetto or the alpha-blocker drug alfuzosin found that the drug had a more rapid onset of action, with 71.8 per cent of men experiencing an increased rate of urinary flow by Day 21 of the trial, compared with 48.4 per cent of those receiving *Serenoa repens*. The irritative score, maximum and average urinary flows, and residual urine volume with both treatments were similar, however. Unfortunately, the trial then ended and *Serenoa* was not given the chance to show its true effects, which would have been expected to continue to show an improvement for several additional weeks if not months.

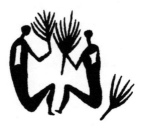

Other Herbal Remedies Used to Treat Prostate Problems

Continental Europe has led the field in natural prostate treatments for many years, and more herbal remedies than conventional drugs are now used to treat prostate symptoms. In Germany, for example, phytotherapy is prescribed for 95 per cent of patients undergoing medical treatment of BPH. In France, natural plant extracts are used by around 40 per cent of men with symptoms that warrant intervention. In Italy, plant extracts represent almost 50 per cent of treatments for BPH, while synthetic drugs such as alpha-blockers and 5-alpha-reductase inhibitors account for only around 5 per cent each of BPH treatments.

Because of the great interest in herbal medicines, around 30 herbal preparations are available throughout Europe[1] for the treatment of prostate problems, most of which are derived from one or more of the following plants:

- Saw Palmetto (*Serenoa repens, Sabal serrulata*)
- Rye pollen (*Secale cereale*)
- Evening primrose (*Oenothera biennis*)

- South African star grass (*Hypoxis rooperi*)
- African prune (*Pygeum africanum*)
- Stinging nettle (*Urtica dioica, Urtica urens*)
- Pumpkin seed (*Cucurbita pepo*)
- Cactus flower extracts
- Bee pollen
- Muira Puama
- Damiana
- Catuaba

Like conventional drugs, herbal extracts have different actions on the prostate gland to improve symptoms. Some shrink or soften the gland to open up the urethra, others relax muscle fibres and reduce spasm of the prostate and bladder, and some damp down inflammation and swelling.

Comparison of these plant extracts shows that they all contain hormone-like substances (phytosterols) such as beta-sitosterol, campesterol, stigmasterol, lupenone, lupeol, fatty acids and flavonoids. It is increasingly thought that the most active ingredient in all of them may be beta-sitosterol, which can also be found in a variety of other plant sources such as soy, pine and spruce tree extracts. A review[2] of four studies in which a total of 519 men took either extracts containing beta-sitosterol or inactive placebo reported that for those taking beta-sitosterol the International Prostate Symptoms Score was reduced by an average of 4.9 points, peak urinary flow rate improved by 3.91 ml/s and residual urinary volume fell by an average of 28.62 ml.

Rye Pollen (*Secale cereale*) and BPH

Extracts from the flower pollen of certain plants, especially rye grass, have also been shown to improve prostate symptoms by reducing prostate swelling, pain, irritation, inflammation, spasm and residual urinary volume, and strengthening urinary flow.

These beneficial effects were first noticed when a Swedish Professor of Urology gave pollen extracts to some of his patients as a convalescent tonic. When the patients told him their prostate symptoms had disappeared, he persuaded the manufacturers of the pollen tonic to investigate further.

Rye pollen extracts are harvested from a variety of rye grass species grown organically in the unpolluted Scania area of southern Sweden. Two different pharmacologically-active fractions are now recognized within the rye extract: a water-soluble fraction (called T60) and a fat-soluble fraction (called GBX) which contains plant hormones (3-β sterols) similar to human oestrogen (oestrone).[3]

Research

A double-blind placebo-controlled study of 60 patients with BPH showed that rye pollen extracts improved prostate symptoms by 69 per cent over six months, compared with only 29 per cent for those taking placebo.[4] Night-time urination (nocturia) decreased significantly by 60 per cent compared with 30 per cent with placebo, and there was a decrease in the amount of urine remaining in the bladder after voiding by 57 per cent (vs 10 per cent). Other symptoms also improved, although these did not reach statistical significance (hesitancy by 47 per cent [vs 29 per cent], urgency by 71 per cent [vs 45 per cent], stopping and starting mid-stream by 52 per cent [vs 33 per cent]). There was also a significant decrease in the diameter of the prostate when measured by ultrasound.

In a trial of 100 patients,[5] natural rye extracts (prescribed for prostatitis) were well tolerated by 97 per cent of patients.

First signs of improvement usually show within three months of treatment, and there is a progressive improvement over a six-month period.

Pollen Extracts and Prostatitis

As well as helping symptoms due to BPH, studies show that rye extracts can help to improve prostate symptoms due to inflammation, irritation and swelling (prostatitis).

An open trial of 15 patients with chronic non-bacterial prostatitis and prostatodynia showed that 13 patients gained complete and lasting relief of symptoms or a marked improvement. Only 2 patients failed to respond.[6]

Another study[7] divided 100 patients with chronic prostatitis and prostatodynia into two groups – those with and without complicating factors such as narrowing of the urinary outlet (urethral stricture, stones in the prostate gland [prostatic calculi] and thickening of the bladder neck [sclerosis]).

In the uncomplicated group, 78 per cent had a favourable response to pollen extract, with 36 per cent being cured of their symptoms and signs. Just over two-fifths (42 per cent) also enjoyed a significant improvement in their urinary flow rate from an average of 15.9 ml/s before treatment to 23.9 ml/s after six months of treatment. The number of pus cells and inflammatory chemicals in the urine after prostate massage was also reduced.

The prostate gland returned to normal size in 15 out of 39 cases, its consistency improved in 37 out of 68 cases, and it was no longer tender on examination in 47 out of 71 cases. These signs worsened in only 5 patients.

In the patients with complications, only 1 patient showed a treatment response. The researchers therefore suggest that any man with prostatitis whose symptoms fail to improve after taking flower pollen extracts for three months should be investigated for suspected complications.

How Rye Pollen Extracts Work

The exact way in which flower pollen extracts work is unknown. Studies suggest they damp down inflammation[8] and inhibit the enzyme 5-alpha-reductase[9] to encourage shrinking of the prostate gland. This activity seems to be present in the fat-soluble fraction.[10]

Rye pollen extracts also have an anti-inflammatory painkilling effect similar to that of aspirin and ibuprofen, as they have been shown to inhibit the enzyme responsible for the production of inflammatory chemicals (cyclo-oxygenase). Extracts also seem to increase the zinc content of the prostate gland. Studies are currently underway to investigate whether pollen extracts interfere with the production or action of growth factors responsible for stimulating the increased growth of prostate cells which occurs in BPH.

Interestingly, pollen extracts have been shown in the laboratory to inhibit the growth of prostate cancer cells.[11] This raises the exciting possibility that treatments derived from pollen extracts may be able to prevent or treat prostate cancer in the future.

No significant side-effects have occurred and, despite being derived from pollen, no allergic reactions were noted even in those highly sensitive to grass pollen. Monitoring of over 3,000 patients in Germany found only three subjects who had what were described as light symptoms of allergy.[12] The reason for low allergenicity is that, during the extraction process, the long-chain chemicals usually associated with allergy are broken down by enzyme action.

Dose

The usual dose is one to two 252-mg tablets daily for up to eight weeks, after which you can reduce to one tablet per day for as long as required. No significant side-effects have been reported. Most men (78 per cent) with prostate problems will notice a favourable response within three months, and there is a progressive improvement over a six-month period.

Evening Primrose (*Oenothera biennis*, *Oenothera lamarckiana*)

The evening primrose has been used as a herbal medicine for centuries by Native Americans. It has proved beneficial for so many ailments that its folk name is 'King's Cure-All'.

The flowers of the evening primrose bloom for only one day, then quickly set seed. It is the seeds of the plant that are one of the richest plant sources of an essential fatty acid known as GLA (gamma linolenic acid – sometimes shortened to gamolenic acid).

Once in the body, GLA enters a series of metabolic reactions that convert it into the hormone-like substances, prostaglandins, which were first discovered in the prostate gland.

Prostaglandins are involved in lots of different reactions, including control of sex drive and sex hormone balance.

The fact that evening primrose oil (EPO) could help prostate problems was first noted when a 69-year-old man was given EPO at a dose of 3 g daily to treat a raised cholesterol level. The cholesterol level reduced and the man also reported that his prostatic symptoms of urinary retention, urgency, frequency and nocturia also improved progressively until he was symptom-free. Three other men with BPH were then also given EPO and their symptoms duly improved, starting from around three months after the onset of treatment. A pilot study showed that before treatment, daytime urinary frequency averaged 14.8 and nocturia 4.8. After taking evening primrose oil for six months, daytime frequency reduced to 9.8 and nocturia to 2.2.

As many as 80 per cent of people are deficient in essential fatty acids, as our diets frequently do not contain optimal amounts of nuts, seeds, wholegrains and green, leafy vegetables. Some GLA can be synthesized from dietary linoleic acid, but this reaction needs an enzyme (delta-6-desaturase) which is easily blocked by a number of factors including eating too much sugar, saturated (animal) fat and trans-fatty acids (as found in margarines), as well as drinking too much alcohol, smoking cigarettes and a dietary deficiency of vitamins and minerals, especially vitamin B_6, zinc and magnesium. The enzyme also becomes less active as we get older.

When you do not get enough essential fatty acids from your diet, your metabolism can make do with the next best fatty acids available (such as those derived from saturated fats), but as a result prostaglandin imbalances are common. Prostaglandins made from other sorts of fat cannot be converted into the prostaglandins made from the EFAs. As a result, inflammatory conditions (such as prostatitis) and sex hormone imbalances, which may contribute to BPH, occur. Evening primrose oil helps to overcome these imbalances and improve prostate symptoms in men, and symptoms of cyclical breast pain in women.

Substances derived from evening primrose oil seem to be a powerful inhibitor of the prostate enzyme 5-alpha-reductase.[13] GLA has also been shown to inhibit the growth of fibrous tissue and, since the growth of fibrous tissue contributes to BPH, this may be another mechanism by which it exerts its beneficial effects.

The action of GLA is boosted by vitamin E, which helps to preserve GLA in the body. It is therefore important to take a supplement containing both GLA and vitamin E, or to take vitamin E capsules at the same time as taking GLA.

Certain vitamins and minerals are also needed during the metabolism of essential fatty acids. These are vitamin C, vitamin B_6, vitamin B_3 (niacin), zinc and magnesium. If you are taking evening primrose oil, you should therefore ensure that your intake of these is adequate.

Evening primrose oil supplements are safe. The only known side-effect of taking too much is mild diarrhoea. The only people who should not take EPO are those who are allergic to it and those with a relatively rare neurological disorder known as temporal lobe epilepsy.

South African Star Grass (*Hypoxis rooperi*)

South African star grass is a rich source of beta-sitosterol, which makes up to 70 per cent of the dried extracts used to treat prostate symptoms. Extracts of the plant are also under investigation for their anti-cancer action in patients with lung tumours. No toxicity has been found even at high doses.

In a randomized, double-blind, placebo-controlled trial[14] of beta-sitosterol extracts obtained from a number of plants, including Star Grass, 177 men with BPH were treated with 130 mg beta-sitosterol for six months. Significant improvements were found, with a reduction of 5.4 points on the International Prostate Symptoms Score (I-PSS – see page 16), an increase in peak urinary flow rates of 4.5 ml/s and a reduction of 33.5 ml in the amount of urine left in the bladder after voiding. The researchers concluded that beta-sitosterol was an effective option in the treatment of BPH.

In a randomized, double-blind, placebo-controlled multicentre study[15] of 200 men with symptoms due to BPH, those given South African star grass extracts (providing 20 mg beta-sitosterol three times a day for six months) showed significant improvements in their symptoms, with a decrease of over 7 on the average International Prostate Symptoms Score (see page 16), an increase in peak urinary flow (from 9.9 to 15.2 ml/s) and a greater than half reduction in the amount of urine left in the bladder after voiding (30.4 instead of 65.8 ml residual urinary volume). These values did not change in the placebo group. No severe side-effects occurred. One patient developed erectile problems and another reported loss of libido after two months.

The results of this trial showed that extracts of South African star grass were at least as effective as drugs commonly prescribed for prostate problems, but without the frequent side-effects which can occur with them.

African Prune (*Pygeum africanum*)

The bark of the evergreen African plum tree is a popular treatment for BPH in Continental Europe, especially France, where it has been used for over 20 years. Extracts are mainly made up of beta-sitosterol and related substances.

Extracts of Pygeum are known to have anti-inflammatory actions and to stop irritable bladder symptoms (see page 8) by damping down overreactivity of the bladder muscle.[16] This suggests it would be helpful for treating symptoms due to both prostatitis and BPH. Some research has also suggested that *Pygeum africanum* extracts have a weak oestrogen effect which may contribute to its ability to reduce markedly the volume of an enlarged prostate gland.[17] It may also inhibit growth factors responsible for overgrowth of prostate fibre cells.

When 18 men with sexual difficulties due to symptoms of either BPH or prostatitis took *Pygeum africanum* extracts (200 mg per day) for 60 days, all showed significant improvement in urinary symptoms and sexual activity, and swelling of the gland around the urethra was also reduced.[18]

In a multicentre study[19] involving 85 men with prostatism in the Czech and Slovak Republics and in Poland, 100 mg per day of *Pygeum africanum* was given for two months. Night-time frequency (nocturia) was reduced by 32 per cent, and average urinary flow rates and urinary volume were also significantly improved and lasted throughout the following month without treatment.

In a double-blind Polish study[20] involving 134 men with BPH, half received a combination of *Pygeum* plus nettle at a standard dose, while the other half received half the normal daily dose. After a month, urinary flow, residual urine and nocturia were significantly reduced in both groups, and the researchers concluded that half-doses were just as safe and effective as the full recommended dose.

Some earlier trials did not produce impressive results, however.

No serious side-effects have been reported.

Stinging Nettle (*Urtica dioica, Urtica urens*)

Stinging nettle is a perennial plant found throughout the world. Nettle roots contain high concentrations of the hormone-like substances such as beta-sitosterol plus fibrous lignans. Its ability to improve urinary symptoms due to BPH (but without shrinking the gland) is a relatively new finding. Nettle extracts also have a beneficial effect on the prostate gland by competing with testosterone to bind with Sex Hormone Binding Globulin (SHBG) in the circulation.[21] As a result, more testosterone is free and active in the circulation and more can be absorbed into the prostate gland. As it is thought that the prostate enlarges in order to absorb more testosterone as levels reduce in later life, this is an exciting finding. Increased levels of freely circulating testosterone also increase sex drive, which can be reduced in men with prostate symptoms. Another possible way in which it works is in reducing the flow of sodium and potassium ions in and out of prostate cells to reduce their metabolism and growth.[22]

Nettle root extracts can also damp down inflammation, and they are used in the treatment of rheumatoid arthritis.[23] They may also be of benefit in treating prostatitis.

Nettle root is often combined with Saw Palmetto berry extracts and with *Pygeum africanum* extracts.

In an observational study[24] involving 419 specialists and 2,080 patients with BPH, a combined extract containing Saw Palmetto berry and nettle root extracts was given. Before and after comparisons showed improvements in both obstructive and irritative symptoms, and results were described as 'very good' or 'good' in over 80 per cent of cases. Less than 1 per cent of men were suspected of having mild side-effects.

In another trial,[25] 40 men with BPH were randomized to receive either a combined extract of Saw Palmetto and stinging nettle or placebo for six months. Neither the researchers nor patients knew which treatment they were receiving. The men then continued taking their supplements for another six months even though the doctors were by then aware which treatment each man was receiving. After the first six months, the International Prostate Symptoms Score (I-PSS – see page 16) improved from 18.6 to 11.1 and urinary flow rates improved from 14.65 ml/s to 17.95 ml/s in those receiving herbal extracts. IPSS only decreased from 19.0 to 17.6 in those on placebo, and urinary flow rates remain virtually unchanged. At the end of the second six months (that is, after 48 weeks treatment) those receiving active herbal supplements showed continued improvement, with a drop in the I-PSS to 9.8 (compared to only 13.3 with placebo) and a further improvement in urinary flow rate to 19.1 ml/s. This would imply that studies to evaluate these herbal remedies should continue for at least one year – some seem happy to finish the trials after three weeks, however, and then to deduce loudly that they do not work!

An interesting trial[26] compared the activity of a combination of Saw Palmetto berry and nettle root extracts against the prescribed drug finasteride.

A total of 548 men were treated for 48 weeks with either two capsules of plant extracts or one capsule of finasteride daily. The results were similar in both groups, with equivalent reductions in urinary flow rate, International Prostate Symptoms Score (I-PSS – see page 16) and increased quality of life. The natural plant extracts proved superior when it came to side-effects, however, with fewer cases of erectile problems and headache.

As mentioned above in the section on *Pygeum africanum*, in a double-blind Polish study[27] involving 134 men with BPH, half received a combination of *Pygeum* plus nettle at standard dose, while the other half received half the normal daily dose. After a month, urinary flow, residual urine and nocturia were significantly reduced in both groups. The researchers concluded that half-doses were just as safe and effective as the full recommended dose.

Side-effects include occasional mild gastrointestinal upsets. Avoid overdosage as this may cause temporary kidney problems.

Pumpkin Seed (*Cucurbita pepo*)

Pumpkin seeds are a popular snack food with a high oil and vitamin E content. The oil is used as a salad oil, but due to its dark green colour and foaminess it cannot be used for cooking.

Studies in rabbits[28] have shown that extracts of the oil could remarkably reduce bladder pressure and increase bladder complaint as well reducing pressure in the urethra. Little recent research seems to have been done on humans, although there is a long tradition of using pumpkin seeds for prostate problems.

Pumpkin seed extracts are often combined with other active ingredients such as Saw Palmetto and zinc to produce supplements aimed at improving prostate health.

Cactus Flower Extracts

Cactus flower extracts are said to help the symptoms of BPH, but there is no published information regarding their use. A laboratory study[29] has shown, however, that cactus flower extracts can inhibit the activity of the prostate enzyme (5-alpha reductase) linked with the development of BPH, which suggests its anecdotal effectiveness is likely to be based on fact.

Bee Pollen

Bee pollen is widely reputed to alleviate symptoms due to BPH and prostatitis, although there is little research to back it up apart from that carried out into rye grass pollens (see pages 59–62). It certainly makes sense that pollens from plants other than rye grass would have a similar action.

Bee pollen is an ultrafine dust made up of sex cells produced on the anthers of male flowers. Bees collect the pollen when foraging for nectar and store it in the hive as food for the young bees. Bee pollen is a very nourishing food, rich in amino acids, carbohydrates, fatty acids, vitamins, minerals – including zinc – and trace elements.

In ancient Greece and Italy, bee pollen was considered a tonic food for those wanting greater energy, vibrancy and zest for life – hence the original use of rye grass pollen as a nutritional tonic before its action in reducing the symptoms of BPH and prostatitis was discovered.

Avoid if you are allergic to bee products or to pollen.

Muira Puama (*Ptychopetalum olacoides*, *P. guyanna*, *Liriosma ovata*)

Muira Puama – popularly known as Potency Wood – is combined with Saw Palmetto in some supplements aimed at increasing sex drive and improving sexual function in men with benign prostatic hyperplasia (BPH). It contains a variety of steroidal plant hormones, including beta-sitosterol – the active prostate-friendly ingredient found in most herbs used to treat BPH – plus lupeol and campestrol.

Muira puama is derived from the wood of a small tree found in the Brazilian rainforest. It has fragrant white flowers with an aroma reminiscent of jasmine. It is principally used by the natives of the Amazon and Orinoco river basins to enhance sexual desire and combat impotence, and is especially helpful where prostate symptoms are also present. It is widely thought to deserve its reputation as a powerful, prosexual supplement which quickly improves libido.

When the Brazilian government researched 120 local remedies used as an aphrodisiac, Muira Puama was one of only three selected for further study, along with Damiana and Catuaba. Researchers are unsure how it works, but it is thought to stimulate sexual desire both psychologically and physically, through a direct action on brain chemicals (dopamine, noradrenaline and serotonin), the stimulation of nerve endings in the genitals and by boosting production/function of sex hormones, especially testosterone.

A clinical study of 262 patients found that Muira Puama was more effective than Yohimbine (a pharmaceutical extract from the bark of the Yohimbe tree, which is an FDA-approved treatment for impotence), with 62 per cent of subjects complaining of lack of sexual desire claiming that Muira Puama had a dynamic effect on their sex lives, while 51 per cent who had erectile dysfunction felt it was of benefit. The researchers suggested that Muira Puama is one of the best herbs for treating erectile dysfunction and lack of libido.

Interestingly, Muira Puama is also said to prevent some types of baldness. As the conversion of testosterone to DHT is linked with both BPH and male pattern baldness, this suggests that it may be able to inhibit the enzyme 5-alpha-reductase, which is responsible for this reaction. As of the present time no research has investigated this possibility.

Muira puama and Saw Palmetto are said to work synergistically together (that is, the two together produce better results than would be expected from the sum of their individual actions).

No serious side-effects have been reported at therapeutic doses.

Damiana (*Turnera diffusa aphrodisiaca*)

Damiana is another herbal supplement that is said to work synergistically with Saw Palmetto in improving male sexual function when BPH is present.

Damiana is a small shrub with aromatic leaves that smell similar to chamomile. It is native to Mexico, Texas, Central America, the northern Caribbean and Namibia, and has a long tradition of use as an aphrodisiac. Its reputation was well established among the Ancient Mayans of Central America, and there is good evidence that it deserves its reputation as a prosexual supplement.

When the Brazilian government researched 120 local remedies used as aphrodisiacs, Damiana was one of only three selected for further study, along with Catuaba and Muira Puama.

The dried leaves and stems of Damiana (gathered during flowering) contain a variety of steroidal plant hormones, including beta-sitosterol which has been shown to be beneficial for treating prostate symptoms. It also contains around 1 per cent volatile oils such as deltacadinene and thymol, responsible for its pros-exual effects. These volatile, aromatic oils gently stimulate the male urinary tract to produce localized tingling and throbbing sensations. Its alkaloids may also boost circulation to the genital area and increase the sensitivity of nerve endings in the clitoris and penis. It also increases circulation to the penis so that erections are firmer and last longer. These combined effects are said to increase sexual desire, enhance sexual pleasure and stimulate sexual performance, especially in men whose erectile difficulties are linked with BPH.

Some herbalists have suggested that the alkaloids in Damiana could have a testosterone-like effect, but there seems to be no research to support this. When drunk as a tea, Damiana produces a mild euphoria and some people use it almost as a recreational drug.

Damiana is usually taken on an occasional basis when needed rather than regularly. Its power as an aphrodisiac is said to be increased when taken in a 1-to-1 mixture with Saw Palmetto berries.

No serious side-effects have been reported from its use. Some evidence suggests that it may reduce iron absorption from the gut, so it should not be used long-term.

Catuaba (*Erythroxylon catuaba*, *Juniperus brasiliensis*, *Anemopaegma mirandum*)

The dried bark of Catuaba – the Brazilian Tree of Togetherness or Tree of Love – is another prosexual supplement that is helpful for older men who have erectile difficulties associated with prostate symptoms.

Catuaba has long been used by the Amazonian Tupi Indians and there is a famous Brazilian saying: 'Until a father reaches 60, the son is his; after that, the son is Catuaba's' – for the supplement is widely used to maintain potency and fertility in older males and to treat male impotence.

Catuaba tree bark contains aromatic resins and non-addictive alkaloids – catuabins – that are distantly related to cocaine. It acts as a sexual stimulant and natural aphrodisiac. It promotes erotic dreams – usually within 5 to 21 days of taking the extracts regularly – followed by increased sexual desire. It also improves peripheral blood flow, which helps to overcome the erectile difficulties that often accompany BPH.

There is no evidence of unwanted side-effects, even after long-term use.

Diet and Lifestyle

CHAPTER FOUR

There is no longer any doubt that you are what you eat. Eating for a healthy heart, circulation and bones has long been accepted. Eating for a healthy prostate gland is a little more revolutionary, perhaps, but likely to become just as important for male health in the future as the new drive towards eating for healthy breasts is for women. The right diet may even protect against prostate cancer by altering the hormonal environment that encourages the formation of prostate cells.

It is estimated that 80 per cent of cancers of the large bowel, breast and prostate are linked with dietary factors.[1] The evidence is now so strong that a muesli-style snack bar rich in protective plant hormones (phytoestrogens) has been launched in the UK (Preva pb), a bread rich in phytoestrogens has been developed in Australia (Burgen), and nutritional supplements designed to 'help maintain a healthy prostate gland' are widely available.

Diet can affect your hormone balance in several ways, through:

- the agricultural chemicals it contains
- the amount of fibre you eat
- the types of fat and fibre you eat

- the natural plant hormones (phytoestrogens) present in your food
- the amount of vitamins, minerals and trace elements you obtain.

Going Organic

Going organic is strongly recommended as part of a healthy prostate eating pro-gramme. Agrochemicals are applied to plants regularly, when the crop is still in its seed form, during germination and throughout its growing cycle. Each non-organic apple, for example, has been dosed around 40 times with up to 100 additives before you eat it. These chemicals do not just lie on the surface of the produce, but are found beneath the skin and sometimes throughout the flesh itself. While some of these chemicals are considered safe to use on crops, the full effects of many on our long-term health, immunity and reproductive system are still not fully understood.

A wide range of agro chemicals such as pesticides, weed-killers, fungicides, fumigants, growth-promoters, growth-retardants and fertilizers have been linked with ill-health. The Environmental Protection Agency in the US considers that 60 per cent of all herbicides, 90 per cent of all fungicides and 30 per cent of all insec-ticides have the potential to cause cancer. Some affect hormone balance and may well play a role in reduced sex drive, reduced sperm count and reduced fertility.

Environmental chemicals (PCBs, dioxins, traces of HRT and contraceptive pills in drinking water, bovine oestrogens in pregnant cows' milk) are now widely implicated in the increased incidence of prostate cancer and rapidly falling sperm count observed in the West.[2] As a result, increasing numbers of people are choosing to use water filters, and to eat organically. Apart from anything else, research shows that organic foods contain, on average, twice the nutrient content of commercially-grown produce. This is partly because they contain less water and more solid matter, but also due to the soils in which they are grown.

By going organic and choosing foods free from growth-promoters, growth-retardants, pesticides, weed-killers, fungicides, fumigants and fertilizers, you are helping to safeguard your future prostate health.

Fibre

Researchers have found that a high-fat, low-fibre diet is associated with relatively high levels of circulating human oestrogen. This is because sex hormones pass from the bile into the gut, from which they are absorbed back into the circulation. This so-called *enterohepatic circulation* helps to maintain relatively high sex hormone levels. If the gut contains dietary fibre residues, however, these mop up a significant amount of sex hormones so that more are excreted and fewer reabsorbed. As a result, oestrogen levels tend to be lower; this is how a high-fibre diet helps to protect against both breast and prostate cancer.

As well as being important for healthy digestion, dietary fibre – or roughage – also binds some of the harmful chemicals found in a non-organic diet so they are more likely to be excreted rather than absorbed.

There are two main types of fibre: soluble and insoluble.

Soluble fibre is important in the stomach and upper intestines, where it slows digestion and absorption to ensure that blood sugar and fat levels rise relatively slowly so that the metabolism can handle nutrient fluctuations more easily.

Insoluble fibre is most important in the large bowel, where it bulks up the faeces, absorbs water and hastens stool excretion. As a result, every gram of fibre you eat adds around 5 g in weight to your stools. The additional weight comes from absorbed water and other substances plus the additional bulk of bacteria (which multiply due to the energy derived by fermenting insoluble fibre). Bacterial fermentation is important for releasing protective plant hormones from the diet – including those found in supplements such as Saw Palmetto and nettle root – and this is another reason why eating a high-fibre diet is important for prostate health.

Fibre also helps to regulate the bowels and to reduce the risk of constipation which can lead to venous congestion and worsen prostatic pain.

Your diet should ideally provide at least 18 g fibre per day – around 40 per cent higher than the current average Western intake. Some experts recommend that we increase fibre intake even more, to at least 30 g daily, although this is best done slowly to give the digestive system time to adapt – otherwise you may develop initial bloating and distension.

The easiest way to increase the amount of fibre in your diet is to eat more unrefined complex carbohydrates, found in foods such as wholemeal bread, cereals, nuts, grains, root vegetables and fruits.

High Fibre

Foods containing 3 g of fibre per 100 g or more are considered high in fibre. Bran-containing breakfast cereals are one of the highest concentrations of dietary fibre.

Bran	provides 40 g fibre per 100-g portion
Dried apricots	18 g per 100 g
Prunes	13 g per 100 g
Brown bread	6 g per 100 g
Walnuts	6 g per 100 g
Peas	5 g per 100 g
White bread	4 g per 100 g
Cooked wholemeal spaghetti	4 g per 100 g
Cooked brown rice	2 g per 100 g

When increasing fibre intake it is also important to ensure a good fluid intake of at least 2 to 3 litres of fluid (preferably water, definitely not coffee or other caffeinated beverages) per day.

Dietary Fats

Dietary fats have received a bad name in the past, but fat is an important source of energy and provides building blocks for healthy cell membranes, nerve function, immunity and for hormonal balance. Ideally, dietary fats should provide between 25 and 30 per cent of daily energy. At present, around 40 per cent of the energy in the Western diet is derived from animal fats, compared with less than 10 per cent in the Far East where the diet is rich in fruits, vegetables and fibre.

Some fats are essential for health, and are therefore known as Essential Fatty Acids (EFAs). Eating a diet containing the right balance of fats is therefore the key.

Dietary oils and fats are made up from a molecule of glycerol to which three fatty acid chains are attached, to form a molecular shape similar to a capital E. The length of the fatty acid chains and whether or not any of their carbon atoms are linked by a double bond are what determines whether the fat is a solid or liquid at room temperature, and also how it is metabolized in the body.

- Fats that contain no double bonds are known as saturated fats.
- Fats with one double bond are monounsaturated.
- Those with two or more double bonds are polyunsaturated.

Most dietary fats contain a blend of saturates, monounsaturates and polyunsaturates. In general, saturated fats tend to be solid at room temperature, while monounsaturated and polyunsaturated fats tend to be oils.

Most dietary saturated fats are of animal origin – this is also the type of fat your body preferentially stores in fatty tissues. Most saturated fat in the typical Western diet is hidden, in that it comes as part of other foods (such as meat, cheese, milk, cakes, cookies and pastries) rather than from frying or spreading fats.

Research,[3,4] suggests that men who follow a typical Western diet high in saturated fat have an increased risk of prostate cancer. The food with the strongest positive link to advanced prostate disease is red meat (beef, pork, lamb, sausages, hamburgers, ham, bacon). This study found no link with the intake of dairy products – except possibly butter. The authors of this study conclude that there is good reason to recommend a lower intake of red meat to reduce the risk of prostate cancer.

It is thought that chemicals produced when meat is cooked (amines) can be absorbed from the intestines to trigger the cell damage linked with cancer. As a word of caution, some experts point out that most of the studies have been carried out in the US, where eating fried and barbecued red meat is more widespread. These studies may not represent our dietary habits in the UK – even so, it seems sensible to cut back on consumption of red meat and to eat more vegetarian meals and oily fish in its place. Anti-cancer guidelines suggest eating no more than 140 g red and/or processed meat per day. Certainly vegetarian men are less likely to develop prostate cancer than those who eat meat.[5]

A study[6] looking at disease and diet trends in 28 countries did find an increased risk of prostate cancer associated with drinking the non-fat portion of milk, which the researchers have suggested is related to its calcium content! This seems unlikely.

Unlike saturated fats, polyunsaturated fatty acids (PUFAs) have spare double bonds which make them highly reactive. They are more susceptible to chemical change through attack by free radicals (see page 90) which produces toxins (lipid peroxides) that have been linked with hardening and furring up of artery walls and an increased risk of cancer.

Polyunsaturated fats (PUFAs) are of two main types:

1 omega-3 PUFAs, derived mainly from fish oils

2 omega-6 PUFAs, derived mainly from vegetable oils.

Your body handles omega-3 and omega-6 oils in different ways. Omega-3 fish oils can be converted into hormone-like chemicals (prostaglandins – so-named because they were originally discovered in the prostate gland) which help to damp down inflammation, while omega-6 PUFAs can be converted into prostaglandins that encourage inflammation. Omega-6 fatty acids have been shown to increase the growth of breast cancer cells in the laboratory, while beneficial omega-3 fatty acids (found, for example, in fish, olive and linseed oils) are known to protect against oestrogen-sensitive tissues such as breast cancer and are likely to protect against prostate cancer as well.

Excess dietary omega-6 PUFAs is believed by some researchers to be linked with an increased risk of chronic inflammatory diseases – such as prostatitis – and possibly an increased risk of some cancers.

The average Western diet currently contains a ratio of omega-6 to omega-3 fats of around 7:1, which is now felt to be far too high. Ideally the balance should be no more than 5:1 and – optimally should be nearer 1:1.

It is worth increasing your intake of nuts, seeds, dark green leafy vegetables and oily fish (such as salmon, herring, mackerel, pilchards, sardines). Aim to eat oily fish (preferably from seas declared to be organic to reduce exposure to pollutants) at least twice a week, if not more. For those who do not like eating fish, fish oil supplements are widely available. Those that are emulsified help to prevent the fishy 'burps' that some people find unpleasant. It is also important to cut back on omega-6 PUFAs (found in margarines, biscuits, cakes, etc.).

Essential Fatty Acids

The essential fatty acids (EFAs) cannot be synthesized in your body from other dietary fats and must therefore come from your food. There are two EFAs:

1 linoleic acid – an omega-6 PUFA

2 linolenic acid – an omega-3 PUFA

In addition, arachidonic acid – an omega-6 PUFA – may be essential if supplies of other EFAs (from which it can be made in the body) are low.

EFAs are found in nuts, seeds, green leafy vegetables, oily fish and whole-grains, or can be taken in supplements such as evening primrose oil. It is esti-mated that as many as 8 out of 10 people do not get enough EFAs from their diet. In addition, metabolic pathways involved in the metabolism of EFAs can be blocked by factors that include excessive intakes of saturated fat, sugar and alcohol, lack of vitamins and minerals, and smoking cigarettes or being under excessive stress.

EFAs act as building blocks for hormones and hormone-like chemicals known as prostaglandins. Lack of EFAs has been linked with a wide range of disease, including BPH and prostatitis.

Evening primrose oil supplements (EPO) are a rich source of gamma-linolenic acid and help to overcome a lack of EFAs in the diet. They are now also known to help protect against BPH and are included in some natural supple-ments designed to improve prostate symptoms (see page 7). EFA supplements are also likely to reduce inflammation in prostatitis.

Dietary Sources of Essential Fatty Acids

- Linoleic acid alone is found in sunflower seeds, almonds, corn, sesame seeds, safflower oil and extra virgin olive oil.

- Linolenic acid alone is found in evening primrose oil, starflower (borage) seed oil and blackcurrant seed oil.

- Both linoleic and linolenic acids are found in rich quantities in walnuts, pumpkin seeds, soybeans, linseed oil, rapeseed oil and flax oil.

- Arachidonic acid is found in many foods (such as seafood, meat, dairy products) and can also be made from linoleic or linolenic acids in the body.

One of the richest sources of the beneficial essential fatty acid GLA (gamma linolenic acid – sometimes shortened to gamolenic acid) is evening primrose oil (see page 62).

Natural Plant Oestrogens

Many plants contain natural chemicals that have a weak, hormone-like action in the human body. These plant hormones, known as phytoestrogens, help to maintain a healthy hormone balance and are strongly believed to play a preventive role in helping to reduce the risk of a number of diseases, including BPH, prostatitis and prostate cancer.

The three main types of phytoestrogens in the diet are isoflavonoids, flavonoids and lignans.

Isoflavonoids are found in members of the pea and bean family such as soya and chickpeas.

Flavonoids are present in high concentrations in many fruits, vegetables – especially apples and onions – and also found in both green and black tea leaves.

Lignans are found mainly in linseed but also in sesame seeds, wholegrain cereals, fruit and vegetables – all of which are widely consumed by Eastern men.

The traditional Japanese diet is low in fat, especially saturated fat, and consists of rice, soy products (such as soybeans, soymeal, tofu) and fish together with legumes, grains and yellow-green vegetables such as cruciferous plants – these include exotic members of the cabbage and turnip families (such as kohlrabi; Chinese leaves). Soy and cruciferous plants are a rich source of isoflavonoids which are then converted into biologically-active hormone-like substances by the intestinal bacteria, especially when the diet is also rich in fibre. Cruciferous vegetables also protect against prostate cancer because they contain a chemical (indole-3-carbinol) needed to metabolize sex hormones in the body more efficiently. Most excitingly of all, researchers have found that the isoflavonoids can damp down the growth of new blood vessels into developing tumours so they do not receive all the blood and oxygen they need to continue developing. As a result, eating 25 g linseed daily can help oestrogen-sensitive tumours to shrink significantly.

In Japan, Asia, the Mediterranean and Latin America the average person consumes 20 to 100 mg of soy isoflavonoids per day. In contrast, the typical Western diet provides only 2 to 5 mg isoflavonoids per day. When the urinary excretion of plant hormones was measured in 10 women and 9 men living in rural Japan, the levels found were exceptionally high.[7] Another study[8] measured the blood concentrations of phytoestrogens in Japanese men and found they were up to 110 times higher than in Finnish male controls.

This is not a genetic effect, as if Japanese people move to the West and follow a typical Western diet, their blood hormone levels and risk of illnesses such as coronary heart disease and cancer quickly become similar to those of the local population. Unfortunately, there are signs that Eastern males who adopt a more Western diet – with increased intakes of total calories, fat and animal protein, and decreased intakes of vegetables and wholegrains – are losing their traditional protection against prostate disease.[9]

Plants Rich in Oestrogen-like Substances

Seeds	almost all, especially linseeds, pumpkin seeds, sesame seeds, sunflower seeds and sprouted seeds (such as alfalfa, mung beans, lentils, red clover, soya beans)
Nuts	especially almonds, cashew nuts, hazelnuts, peanuts, walnuts and nut oils
Wholegrains	almost all, especially corn, buckwheat, millet, oats, rye, wheat
Fresh fruits	apples, avocados, bananas, mangoes, papayas, rhubarb
Dried fruits	especially dates, figs, prunes and raisins
Vegetables	dark green leafy vegetables (such as broccoli, Bok choi, spinach, spring greens, watercress), celery, fennel and exotic members of the cruciferous family (such as Chinese leaves, kohl rabi)
Legumes	especially soy beans and soy products (such as tofu, tempeh, miso,

tamari), chickpeas, lentils

Herbs	especially angelica, chervil, chives, garlic, ginger, horseradish, nutmeg, parsley, rosemary and sage
Honey	especially that made from wild flowers

Bread (such as Burgen) and muesli-style bars (such as Preva pb, Wallaby bars) fortified with soya and linseed to make them rich in natural plant oestrogens are now widely available in supermarkets and health food stores.

The Dietary Importance of Soya Beans

Soya beans are a rich source of isoflavonoids – the plant hormones that have a similar structure to human oestrogen and corticosteroid hormones produced by the adrenal glands. The principle isoflavonoids found in soy are daidzein, genistein and glycitein. These isoflavonoids are 500 times less active than the main human oestrogen, oestradiol, but can still bind to oestrogen receptors in the body. These weak oestrogens are helpful in normalizing oestrogen balance when levels are either high or low. This may seem confusing, but is easily explained.

When oestrogen levels are low (such as at the time of the menopause in women), these weak plant hormones can provide enough oestrogen activity to reduce the severity of hot flushes and night sweats.

When problems are linked to excessively high oestrogen levels, however, the weaker plant hormones basically compete with the stronger oestrogens for landing sites (receptors) on oestrogen-sensitive tissues such as the breasts and prostate gland. This reduces the effect of the stronger oestrogens by replacing it with much weaker activity. Overall, oestrogen exposure is therefore significantly reduced. This is one way in which the plant hormones found in Saw Palmetto (such as beta-sitosterol) produce their beneficial effect in BPH, although it also has other actions such as greatly reducing the number of oestrogen receptors present (see page 87).

Recently, genistein was found to decrease the growth of both BPH and prostate cancer cells in the laboratory,[10] which the researchers suggested showed that the genistein found in soy has the potential to be used as a treatment for both BPH and prostate cancer in the future.

Phytoestrogens also reduce the effects of human oestrogens in the body by stimulating the production of Sex Hormone Binding Globulin (SHBG), which binds oestrogen in the circulation so that the oestrogen is taken out of action.[11] As it is only free oestrogen that is able to interact with cell receptors, plant hormones reduce the tissue stimulation that can occur from natural human oestrogen, and possibly from environmental pollutants, too.

By reducing oestrogen exposure, soya isoflavonoids can protect against a number of cancers, including prostate cancer. Isoflavonoid phytoestrogens are also thought to have a direct effect on tumour cell growth, and it has been estimated that eating just one bowl of miso soup (made from fermented soya beans) per day may reduce the risk of stomach cancer, for example, by more than 30 per cent.

Genistein is now also thought to protect against prostate cancer by interfering with the way hormones and growth factors interact in the prostate gland to stimulate abnormal growth of prostate cancer cells.[12]

Isoflavonoids also have an antioxidant action and have been found to reduce inflammation. They may also have a protective action against prostatitis.

A daily intake of at least 50 mg isoflavonoids is recommended. Sixty grams of soy protein provides 45 mg isoflavonoids.

Eating one bar of Preva pb (which contains soya, linseed, rye bran, oats, rice, wheat flakes and apples) can change blood levels of the isoflavonoid genistein from an average of 36 ng/ml to 93 ng/ml — much closer to that of a Japanese male — within six hours.

Tomatoes

A high intake of tomatoes seems to protect against prostate cancer. Tomatoes are a rich source of a red carotenoid pigment known as lycopene which is a powerful antioxidant. Tomato extracts have been shown to be concentrated in a variety of organs, including the prostate gland.

Research suggests there is a strong inverse relationship between blood levels of lycopene and the risk of prostate cancer. Out of 72 different studies looking at this relationship, 57 found that the higher the intake and blood levels of lycopene, the lower the risk of prostate cancer.[13] One study[14] found that men with the highest lycopene levels were up to 60 per cent less likely to develop prostate cancer than those with the lowest blood levels. Laboratory experiments suggest that when lycopene and vitamin E act together, prostate cancer cells are stopped from growing and multiplying by as much as 90 per cent.[15] When 12 men with prostate cancer were compared with 12 similar men without prostate cancer, blood lycopene levels were 44 per cent lower and prostate tissue lycopene was 78 per cent lower in those with the disease compared with those without.[16] Increasing your intake of tomatoes may well reduce your risk of developing or worsening prostate cancer.

Dietary Antioxidants

Eastern men eat many more yellow, orange, red and green vegetables than Western males. These are rich sources of antioxidant vitamins (E, C and beta-carotene) which help to protect against most cancers, including that of the prostate gland.[17] Their protection is believed to come from their ability to neutralize highly reactive molecular fragments known as free radicals.

A free radical is an unstable molecular fragment that carries a minute, negative electrical charge in the form of a spare electron. It tries to lose this charge by passing on its spare electron during collisions with other molecules and cell structures. This process is known as oxidation. Oxidation usually triggers a harmful chain reaction in which electrons are passed from one molecule to another with damaging results.

Body proteins, fats, cell membranes and genetic material (DNA) are constantly under attack from free radicals, with each cell undergoing an estimated 100,000 free radical oxidations per day – the number is twice as high in smokers. These collisions and chain reactions are one of the main causes of the genetic damage (mutations) leading to cancer.

Free radicals are continuously produced in the body as a result of:

- normal metabolic reactions
- muscle contraction during exercise

- smoking cigarettes

- drinking excessive amounts of alcohol

- exposure to environmental pollutants

- exposure to x-rays

- exposure to UVA sunlight, especially if sunburned

- taking some drugs – especially antibiotics or paracetamol.

Dietary antioxidants are the body's main defence against free radical attack. They quickly neutralize the negative charge on a free radical before it can trigger a chain reaction.

Vitamin E is an antioxidant that has been shown to reduce significantly the risk of prostate cancer. When given to male smokers, researchers found a 32 per cent decreased risk of developing prostate cancer in men taking 50 mg vitamin E daily, compared to men not receiving vitamin E in a trial that involved over 29,000 men.[18] In addition, the risk of dying from prostate cancer was reduced by 41 per cent in those taking vitamin E. This suggests that the antioxidant vitamin E is highly protective against prostate cancer in male smokers. Unfortunately, those given supplements of beta-carotene (20 mg daily) showed a 23 per cent increased risk of prostate cancer. This result needs further investigation.

Vitamins and Minerals

It is estimated that only 1 in 10 people get all the vitamins and minerals they need from their diet. Even if only one micronutrient is in short supply it can affect hormone balance and may make prostate symptoms worse. It is therefore important that your intake of nutrients is balanced. If taking a vitamin and mineral supplement, for example, it's best to take one supplying around 100 per cent of the recommended daily amount (RDA) of as many vitamins and minerals as possible. The following table shows which vitamins and minerals are especially important for prostate health.

Micronutrient (Adult EC RDA – where set)	Sex hormone function	Food Sources
Vitamin A (800 mcg)	Regulates sexual growth, development and reproduction by switching on genes in response to sex hormone triggers. Essential for the production of sex hormones, including oestrogen and testosterone. Powerful antioxidant.	Animal and fish livers, kidneys, eggs, milk, cheese, yoghurt, butter, oily fish, meat, margarine. As beta-carotene: dark green leafy vegetables and yellow-orange fruits.
Vitamin B_{12} (1 mcg)	Found in prostate secretions.	Liver, kidney, oily fish – especially sardines, red meat, white fish, eggs, dairy products.
Vitamin C (60 mg)	Antioxidant which provides important protection against	Citrus fruits, blackcurrants, guavas, kiwi fruit, green

	free radical attack. Its anti-inflammatory action is likely to be beneficial in prostatitis.	peppers, strawberries, green sprouting vegetables.
Vitamin E (10 mg)	Plays a key role in the manufacture of sex hormones and protects them from oxidation and degradation. Powerful antioxidant. May help to prevent prostatitis.	Oily fish, fortified margarine and dairy products, liver, eggs.
Boron	Needed for the production of sex hormones.	Fruit and vegetables.
Copper (1.1 mg)	Found in prostate secretions.	Shellfish and crustaceans, yeast, olives, nuts, pulses, wholegrains, green vegetables.
Magnesium (300 mg)	Most magnesium found in semen is derived from prostate secretions. The prostate has one of the highest magnesium concentrations found in body tissues.	Soya beans, nuts, yeast, wholegrains, brown rice, seafood, meat, eggs, dairy products, bananas, green leafy vegetables.
Manganese	Found in prostate secretions.	Black tea, wholegrains, nuts, seeds, fruit, eggs, green leafy vegetables, offal, shellfish, dairy products.

Phosphorus (800 mg)	Found in prostate secretions.	Dairy products, yeast, soya beans, nuts, wholegrains, eggs, poultry, meat and fish.
Potassium	Most potassium found in semen is derived from prostate secretions.	Fresh fruit and vegetables, low-salt substitutes.
Selenium	Essential for the synthesis of prostaglandins and sex hormones.	Brazil and other nuts, broccoli, mushrooms, cabbage, radishes, onions, garlic, celery, wholegrains, yeast, seafood, offal.
Zinc (15 mg)	The zinc found in semen is derived almost exclusively from prostate secretions. The prostate has the highest zinc content of all body tissues.	Red meat (especially offal), seafood (especially oysters), yeast, wholegrains, pulses, eggs, cheese.

Zinc

Zinc is especially important for prostate health, and its concentration in the prostate is much higher than in any other body tissue. It is an important co-factor for over a hundred metabolic enzymes. It forms an integral part of the enzyme which switches on particular genes in response to hormone triggers, and plays a major role in the sensitivity of the prostate gland to circulating sex hormones.

In some parts of the world, dietary zinc deficiency is common and results in delayed male puberty. Studies suggest that low intakes of dietary zinc (less than 5 mg per day) are also associated with low testosterone levels.[19] This increases relative exposure to oestrogens and may increase the risk of prostate problems. Intakes of at least 10 mg zinc per day are needed to maintain prostate health. The recommended daily amount for adults is 15 mg per day.

Zinc is so important for sperm health that each ejaculate contains around 5 mg zinc – one-third of the daily requirement. Men who are sexually active are therefore at risk of zinc deficiency. Lack of zinc is associated with an increased risk of prostatitis,[20] as zinc levels are low in inflamed prostate tissues. Recently it was discovered that measuring the zinc content of prostate biopsy samples could help to determine whether or not prostate cancer was present,[21] as prostate cancer cells also lose their ability to concentrate zinc – so levels are much lower in abnormal tissue.

One of the earliest symptoms of zinc deficiency is loss of taste sensation. This can be tested for by obtaining a solution of zinc sulphate (5 mg/5 ml) from a chemist. Swirl a teaspoonful in your mouth. If the solution seems tasteless, zinc deficiency is likely. If the solution tastes furry, of minerals or slightly sweet, zinc levels are borderline. If it tastes strongly unpleasant, zinc levels are normal.

Selenium

Selenium is a mineral that has important antioxidant actions. Research suggests that men taking a supplement of 200 mcg selenium had one-third the risk of prostate cancer compared with men receiving inactive placebo.[22] As a result, a prospective study was designed in which the association between selenium levels in toenail clippings was compared with the future diagnosis of prostate cancer over a five-year period. Toenail clippings were collected from over 33,700 men and those with the highest levels of selenium were found to be 65 per cent less likely to develop prostate cancer than those with low levels.

Vitamin D

Vitamin D has been found to reduce the growth and division of prostate cancer cells in the laboratory. Researchers feel that vitamin D may be a useful treatment for prostate cancer in the future and that its actions need further investigation.[23]

Dietary Tips for Male Prostate Health

1 Go organic and avoid exposure to plastics, which contain potentially harmful chemicals. Wrap food in greaseproof rather than cling film and use ceramic dishes for freezing foods rather than plastic ones.

2 Eat more fibre: aim for at least 30 g per day.

3 Follow a low-fat diet.

4 Obtain a balance of dietary fats: eat more omega-3 and fewer omega-6 polyunsaturated fatty acids.

5 Reduce intake of saturated fat – especially red meat.

6 Eat more oily fish.

7 Increase your intake of unrefined carbohydrates such as whole-grains.

8 Eat more fruit and vegetables, especially cruciferous vegetables

such as broccoli. In the UK, we eat less than half the amount of fruit and vegetables per day eaten by Mediterranean races who have a low risk of cancer. Ideally we need to at least double our intake. At least five servings of fresh fruit, vegetables or salad stuff per day – and preferably 7 to 10 servings daily.

9 Increase fruit intake by drinking fruit juices and eating fresh and dried fruit as snacks.

10 Eat more nuts and seeds for essential fatty acids – aim for a tablespoon of linseed daily. Linseed can be eaten whole, sprinkled on salads or ground and mixed with fruit juice, cottage cheese, fromage frais or yoghurt.

11 Eat more soya-based foods. Soya is hard to include in a Western diet, so eat soya/linseed bars (available in health food shops) to increase your intake of phytoestrogens. Also try using soya flakes instead of nuts as a snack. If you don't like soya, eat plenty of pulses such as chickpeas, kidney, black-eyed peas or mung beans.

12 Eat more tomatoes – try roasting a kilogram when the oven is on and using them to make soup.

13 Ensure a good intake of zinc, found in seafood – especially oysters – wholegrains, bran, pumpkin seeds, garlic and pulses.

14 Consider taking antioxidant supplements.

15 Reduce your salt intake.

16 Avoid or limit your intake of tea (but see below), coffee and other caffeinated drinks.

17 Reduce your intake of sugar and use fruit (such as puréed rasp-
berries) as a sweetener instead.

18 Avoid convenience, pre-processed foods and additives – eat home-
made meals as often as possible.

19 Drink plenty of fluids, especially mineral or filtered water.

20 Drink more tea – made from either green or black tea-leaves for
their flavonoid content.

21 Drink less milk.

22 Consider taking supplements containing vitamins C, E, selenium,
zinc and possibly vitamin D.

23 Consider taking evening primrose oil supplements.

Lifestyle Changes for Prostate Health

A number of lifestyle changes can reduce your risk of prostate problems such as
BPH, prostatitis and prostate cancer.

Stop Smoking

Smoking has an adverse effect on hormone balance in the body and is also
linked with an increased risk of cancer generally. Some studies show a definite link
between smoking and prostate cancer, but others do not. Interestingly, it seems that
men who smoke are less likely to need surgery for BPH than those who do not –
probably because smoking lowers levels of oestrogen hormone.[24] This is *not* a reason
to continue smoking, however! There is a definite relationship between currently
smoking 35 or more cigarettes per day and the risk of BPH compared with men

who have never smoked.[25] If you do smoke, it is worth making the effort to stop to reduce your risk of cancer, including possibly that of the prostate gland.

Go Easy on the Alcohol

Although a moderate intake of alcohol is beneficial for the circulation and helps to reduce the risk of coronary heart disease, sadly there is a direct link between the amount of alcohol we drink and the risk of cancer. Research involving around a third of a million women followed up for 11 years showed that over the normal consumption range, the risk of breast cancer increased by around 9 per cent with every drink. As a result, women who drank up to 5 units of alcohol per day were over 40 per cent more likely to develop breast cancer at some time in their lives than those not drinking any alcohol at all. The researchers therefore stated that, among women who consume alcohol regularly, reducing alcohol consumption is a potential means to reduce their risk of breast cancer.

A similar relationship is likely to hold true for men and prostate cancer. Anti-cancer guidelines suggest drinking no more than 3 units of alcohol per day for men (and 2 units a day for women). Some men with prostatitis also find that sensitivity to alcohol (and occasionally caffeine) can trigger an attack of prostate pain – in which case it is worth avoiding these.

Lose Any Excess Weight

Fatty tissues convert circulating sex hormones into oestrogen, so that men who are overweight have higher oestrogen levels than those who are a healthy weight for their height. The link between weight gain and breast cancer in women is well established – gaining more than 25 kg in weight during adulthood more than doubles the risk of breast cancer in some women, especially those who were initially underweight. A similar relationship is likely to hold true for men and prostate cancer. Do all you can to prevent middle-aged spread, and if you have put on weight, aim to get back to a healthy weight for your height by following a prostate-friendly diet and increasing the amount of exercise you take.

Exercise

Research[26] shows that men who are more physically active are significantly less likely to develop lower urinary tract symptoms due to BPH. Men who walked for two to three hours per week were 25 per cent less likely to develop BPH than those who did little walking. Brisk, aerobic exercise (such as brisk walking, jogging, cycling, swimming, dancing) helps to lower oestrogen levels and can therefore help to reduce the risk of prostate cancer. For optimum health, aim to exercise enough to raise your pulse and leave you slightly breathless, for 20 to 30 minutes at least 5 times a week and preferably every day. It is important not to exercise on a full bladder, however, as this is one possible cause of prostatitis.

Exercises to Reduce Pelvic and Prostate Congestion

Symptoms of prostate enlargement due to poor circulation, congestion or swelling may be helped by the following exercises:

- Alternate sitting in hot and cold water – use a bidet or large bowl.
- Practise the Deer exercise – devised by the ancient Chinese – to strengthen the anal muscles and massage the prostate gland:
  - Sit, stand or lie, which ever you find most comfortable.
  - Squeeze your anal muscles together tightly and hold for as long as is comfortable.
  - Relax for a minute or two then repeat as many times as is comfortable.
- Try the yoga position known as Baddha Konasana (Bound angle or Cobbler's) posture. This drains pelvic congestion and is used by Indian shoe-menders, who rarely develop prostate problems
  - Sit on the floor.
  - Bring the soles of your feet together, pulling your heels up as close to your groin as possible.
  - Keep your back and shoulders straight and your head up.
  - Try to let your knees sink towards the ground so that the soles of your feet are flat against each other.
  - Hold your ankles and relax for as long as is comfortable.

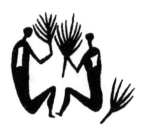

Glossary

Androgen
A male hormone that produces masculinization in either sex

Benign prostatic hyperplasia (BPH)
Non-cancerous increase in the size of the prostate gland due to an increase in the number of cells present

Carcinoma
A type of cancer

Contraindication
A factor that makes it unwise to prescribe a certain drug because of the potential for serious side-effects

Cross-over trial
Study in which groups of patients take a trial substance, then cross over and, after a wash-out period, taken another trial substance (or placebo). This allows the effects of active substances (plus or minus placebo) to be assessed in all volunteers.

Cystoscopy
Direct visual examination of the lower urinary tract using a viewing device known as a cystoscope that is inserted into the urinary passage under general anaesthetic

Dihydro-testosterone
A powerful androgen formed when the enzyme 5-alpha-reductase acts on testosterone hormone

Double-blind trial
A study in which neither the volunteers nor the researchers

know which person is using which treatment until the code is cracked after the trial has ended. Removes the possibility of experimental bias.

Drug   A substance that affects living organisms and is used to prevent, diagnose, relieve or cure a medical problem

Dysuria   Pain or discomfort on passing water

Erectile Dysfunction Difficulty in obtaining or maintaining an erection

5-alpha-reductase Prostate enzyme that converts testosterone hormone to DHT

Frequency   Having to pass urine more frequently than normal

Haematuria   Presence of blood in the urine

Herbalist   Someone who uses natural plant substances to help relieve the symptoms of a disease

Hesitancy   Difficulty or delay in starting to pass urine

Hyperplasia   Increase in the number of cells present in a tissue or organ, causing an overall increase in size

Intermittency   Stopping and starting when passing urine rather than producing a continuous stream

Multicentre Trial A study in which volunteers are recruited and followed-up at more than one centre. Allows a broader section of the population to be involved.

Nocturia   Having to get up at night to pass urine

Phytotherapy   The use of plant (herbal) extracts for healing

Placebo   An inactive substance identical in appearance to the material being researched. It is given as an unbiased control to evaluate the effectiveness of the material being researched.

Prospective study A type of epidemiological study that looks at events in one or more populations and follows them over a period of time to see what statistically-significant differences develop. More likely than a retrospective study to yield scientifically valid results.

Prostate specific antigen (PSA) A protein (enzyme) found only in the prostate gland which may be used as a marker to predict the likely presence of prostate cancer

Randomized study A study design in which volunteers have an equal chance of ending up in either the treatment or the placebo (control) group

Stroma A tissue that forms the framework and covering of an organ

Testosterone The main male (androgenic) hormone

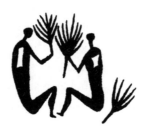

Sources of Information

PROSTATE HELP ASSOCIATION (PHA)

Langworth

Lincoln LN3 5DF

A non-profit-making charity developed to collate information on prostate problems and treatments. Please enclose a large SAE when writing.

PROSTATE RESEARCH CAMPAIGN UK

36 The Drive

Northwood

Middlesex HA6 1HP

Provides leaflets, promotes education and finances research. Please send two first-class stamps for initial information.

PROSTATE CANCER CHARITY

Du Cane Road

London W12 0NN

Confidential helpline: 020 8383 1948

107

IMPERIAL CANCER RESEARCH FUND

PO Box 123

Lincoln's Inn Fields

London WC2A 3PX

Provides information and carries out research into the causes, pre-
vention, treatment and cure of cancer.

Helplines

SMOKERS' QUITLINE

020 7487 3000 (9.30 a.m. – 5.30 p.m. daily)

MEN'S HEALTH MATTERS ADVICELINE

020 8995 4448 (Mon–Fri 6 p.m. to 8 p.m.)

FREEPHONE CANCER INFORMATION HELPLINE

0800 132905

EFAMOL (EVENING PRIMROSE OIL) INFORMATION LINE

01483 570248

PREVA PB CUSTOMER INFORMATION LINE

0870 240 2618

Product Manufacturers and Suppliers

THE NUTRI CENTRE

The Hale Clinic

7 Park Crescent

London W1N 3HE

Tel: 020 7436 5122

Supplies by mail order many of the herbal, vitamin and mineral supplements mentioned in this book.

BRITANNIA HEALTH PRODUCTS LTD

41–51 Brighton Road

Redhill

Surrey RH1 6YS

Tel: 01737 773741

Fax: 01737 762672

Supply: ProstaBrit rye pollen extracts

EFAMOL LTD

Weyvern House

Weyvern Park

Portsmouth Road

Peasmarsh

Guildford

Surrey GU3 1NA
Tel: 01483 304441
Fax: 01483 304437
Order Line: 0800 318545

Supply: Efaprost (Evening primrose oil, Saw Palmetto, beta-sitos-terol) for men, Efamol (Evening primrose oil)

FUTUREBIOTICS

Hauppauge, New York
Tel: 1-800-FOR-LIFE
website: www.futurebiotics.com

Supply: Male Power (male energizing formula containing Korean ginseng, wild oats, Saw Palmetto, Fo Ti, Schisandra, deer antler, bee pollen, Siberian ginseng, wild yam, astragalus, black cohosh, ginger, Royal Jelly and glandular extracts)

HEALTH & DIET COMPANY

Europa Park
Radcliffe
Manchester M26 1GG
Tel: 01204 707420
Fax: 01204 792238

Supply: FSC-Herbcraft ranges (tinctures & capsules), Formula 600 Plus for Men (including zinc, vitamin B_6, copper, Saw Palmetto,

Pygeum africanum and Pumpkin powder, cayenne and amino acids),
Ginseng & Saw Palmetto for Men Tincture, Saw Palmetto Plus
Tincture & Tablets, Damiana, and nettles

HERBAL ALTERNATIVE LABORATORIES LTD

Lime Tree House

Lime Tree Walk

Sevenoaks

Kent TN13 1YH

Tel: 01732 746604

Fax: 01732 465500

Order number at JEM Marketing: 01483 204417

email: herbal_labs@hotmail.com

Supply: Herbal V (containing Muira Puama)

KORDEL HEALTHCARE LTD

Bradford

West Yorks

Tel: 01274 488511

KORDEL (AUSTRALIA) PTY LTD

102 Bath Road

Kirrawee

NSW

HEALTH FOODS INTERNATIONAL LTD

9 Canon Place

Pakuranga

Auckland

> *Supply:* Zest for Men (containing zinc and other vitamins, minerals and trace elements, Damiana, Siberian ginseng, oyster extract, sarsaparilla, Saw Palmetto and cayenne)

LICHTWER PHARMA UK LTD/MEDIC HERB

Regency House

Mere Park

Dedmere Road

Marlow

Bucks SL7 1FJ

Tel: 01628 487780

Fax: 01628 487781

> *Supply:* Sabalin (standardized Saw Palmetto)

LIFE ENHANCEMENT PRODUCTS INC

1340 Industrial Ave

Suite A

Petaluma CA 94952

Toll Free: 1-800-543-3873

Outside US Tel: 1-707 762 6144

Fax: 1-769 8016

website: www.life-enhancement.com

Supply: Saw Palmetto

LIFE PLUS EUROPE LTD

Martin House

Howard Road

Eaton Socon

Cambs PE19 3ET

Tel: 01480 477230

Fax: 01480 403772

LIFE PLUS USA

Box 3749

Batesville AR 72503

Tel 800-572-8446

Supply: Prostate Formula (Saw Palmetto, Jatoba and Pau d'Arco)

NATURE'S REMEDIES LTD

15 Little End Road

Eaton Socon

Cambridgeshire PE19 3JH

Tel 01480 403768

Fax: 01480 403757

Supply: Male Plus Amazon Formula for Men (including Muira Puama, Catuaba, Damiana and Sarsaparilla), Evening Primrose Oil

QUEST VITAMINS LTD

8 Venture Way

Aston Science Park

Birmingham B7 4AP

Tel: 0121 359 0056

Fax: 0121 359 0313

email: info@questvitamins.co.uk

Supply: Saw Palmetto

RIO TRADING

2 Centenary Estate

Brighton

East Sussex BN2 4AW

Tel: 01273 570987

Supply: Catuaba

SOLGAR VITAMINS LTD

Aldbury

Tring

Herts HP23 5PT

Tel: 01442 890355

Fax: 01442 890366

Supply: Gold Label Range (Saw Palmetto, bee pollen)

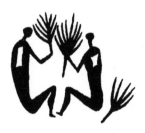

References

SAW PALMETTO

Introduction

1. A C Buck, 'Phytotherapy for the prostate', *British Journal of Urology* 78 (1996): 325–6

2. Ibid.

3. Ibid.

4. F Bracher, 'Phytotherapy of BPH', *Urologe A* 36.1 (1997): 10–17

Chapter 1

1. W M Garraway *et al.*, 'High prevalence of BPH in the community', *Lancet* 338 (1991): 469–71

2. H Weisser and M Krieg, 'BPH – the outcome of age-induced alteration of androgen-estrogen balance?' *Urologe A* 36.1 (1997): 3–9

3. K Suzuki *et al.*, 'Endocrine environment of BPH: prostate size and volume are correlated with serum estrogen concentrations', *Scand J Urol Nephol* 29.1 (1995): 65–8

4. A Zisman *et al.*, 'Autoantibodies to PSA in patients with BPH', *J Urol* 154.3 (1995): 1052–5

5. W G Rober, 'The etiology of BPH', *Med Hypotheses* 50.1 (1998): 61–5

6. G Bedalov *et al.*, 'Prostatitis in BPH: a histological, bacteriological and clinical study', *Acta Med Croatica* 48.3 (1994): 105–9

7. B R Oh *et al.*, 'Association of BPH with male pattern baldness', *Urology* 51.5 (1998): 744–8

8. W M Garraway, 'Impact of previously unrecognised BPH on the daily activities of middle-aged and elderly men', *BJ Gen Pract* 43 (1993): 318–21

9. ProstaBrit, *Sex in Later Life Survey* (MORI, 1993)

10. S J Frankel *et al.*, 'Sexual dysfunction in men with lower urinary tract symptoms', *J Clin Epidemiol* 51.8 (1998): 677–85

11. M V Barry *et al.*, 'The American urological association symptom index for benign prostatic hyperplasia', *J Urol* 148 (1992): 1549–57

12. D J Shore, 'Managing BPH: The shared-care initiative', *Geriatric Medicine* (January 1994): 11–12.

13. P K Grover and M I Resnick, 'Analysis of prostatic fluid: evidence for the presence of a prospective marker for prostatic cancer', *Prostate* 26.1 (1995): 12–18.

14. Carter H Ballentine *et al.*, 'Longitudinal evaluation of PSA levels in men with and without prostate disease', *JAMA* 267 (1992): 2215–20

15. H Kawashima *et al.*, 'A case of giant prostatic calculi', *Hinyokika*

Kiya 38.7 (1992): 853–5

16. Bedalov *et al.*, 'Prostatitis in BPH: a histological, bacteriological and clinical study', *Acta Med Croatica* 48.3 (1994): 105–9

17. K Griffiths *et al.*, 'Phytoestrogens and diseases of the prostate gland', *Ballieres Clin Endocrinol Metab* 12.4 (1998): 625–47

18. D Grignon and W Sakr, 'BPH: is it a premalignant lesion?' *In Vivo* 8.3 (1994): 415–18

19. D G Bostwick *et al.*, 'The association of BPH and cancer of the prostate', *Cancer* 70.1 (suppl; 1992): 291–301

20. G D Steinberg *et al.*, 'Family history and the risk of prostate cancer', *Prostate* 17.4 (1990): 337–47

21. Yu *et al.*, 'Comparative epidemiology of cancers of the colon, rectum, prostate and breast in Shanghai, China versus the US', *Int. J. Epidemiol* 20.1 (1991): 76–81

22. Meares and Sant, *Differential Diagnosis of Prostate Disorders* (Gower Medical Publishing, 1992), 26–8

Chapter 2

1. T J Wilt *et al.*, 'Saw Palmetto extracts for treatment of BPH. A systematic review', *JAMA* 280.18 (1998): 1604–9

2. D Bach *et al.*, 'Phytopharmaceutical and synthetic agents in the treatment of BPH', *Phytomedicine* 3.4 (1996): 309–13

3. G L Plosker and R N Brogden, 'Serenoa repens: A review of its pharmacology and therapeutic efficacy in BPH', *Drugs & Ageing*

9.5 (1996): 379–95

4. C Casarosa *et al.*, 'Lack of effects of a lyposterolic extract of Serenoa repens on plasma levels of testosterone, FSH and LS', *Clin Ther* 10.5 (1988): 585–8

5. S Delos *et al.*, 'Testosterone metabolism in primary cultures of human prostate epithelial cells and fibroblasts', *J Steroid Biochem Mol Biol* 55.3–4 (1995): 375–83

6. G Strauch *et al.*, 'Comparison of finasteride and Serenoa repens in the inhibition of 5-alpha reductase in healthy male volun teers', *Eur Urol* 26.3 (1994): 247–52

7. C Iehle *et al.*, 'Human prostatic steroid 5-alpha-reductase iso-forms – a comparative study of selective inhibitors', *J Steroid Biochem Mol Biol* 54 (1995): 273–9

8. J Weisser *et al.*, 'Effects of sabal serrulata extract IDS89 and its subfractions on 5-alpha-reductase activity in human BPH', *Prostate* 28.5 (1996): 300–306

9. S Delos *et al.*, 'Inhibition of basic 5-alpha-reductase (type 1) detected in DU 145 cells', *J Steroid Biochem* 48 (1994): 347–52

10. S Delos *et al.*, 'Testosterone metabolism in primary cultures of human prostate epithelial cells and fibroblasts', *J Steroid Biochem Mol Biol* 55.3–4 (1995): 375–83

11. F Di Silverio *et al.*, 'Effects of long-term treatment with Serenoa repens on the concentrations and regional distribution of androgens and epidermal growth factor in BPH', *Prostate* 37.2

(1998): 77–83.

12. G L Plosker and R N Brogden, 'Serenoa repens: A review of its pharmacology and therapeutic efficacy in BPH', *Drugs & Ageing* 9.5 (1996): 379–95

13. C Sultan *et al.*, 'Inhibition of androgen metabolism and binding by a liposterolic extract of serenoa repens B in human foreskin fibroblasts', *J Steroid Biochem* 20 (1984): 515–19

14. M Briley *et al.*, 'Inhibitory effect of Permixon on testosterone 5-alpha-reductase activity of the rat ventral prostate', *Br J Pharmacol* 83 (1984): 401P

15. F Di Silverio *et al.*, 'Evidence that Serenoa repens extract displays an antiestrogenic activity in prostatic tissue of BPH patients', *Eur Urol* 21 (1992): 309–14

16. M Goepel *et al.*, 'Saw palmetto extracts potently and noncompetitively inhibit human alpha1-adrenoceptors in vitro', *Prostate* 38.3 (1999): 208–15

17. M M Christiansen and R C Bruskewitz, 'Clinical manifestations of BPH and the indications for therapeutic intervention', *Urol Clin North Am* 17 (1990): 509–16

18. M Gutierrez *et al.*, 'Spasmolytic activity of a lipidic extract from Sabal serrulata fruits: further study of the mechanisms underlying this activity', *Planta Med* 62.6 (1996): 507–11

19. W Breu *et al.*, 'In vitro antagonists of cyclo-oxygenase and 5-lipoxygenase metabolism' *Arzneim-Forsch Drug Res* 42.4

(1992): 547–51

20. M Paubert-Braquet *et al.*, 'Effect of the lipidosterolic extract of Serenoa repens and its major components on basic fibroblast growth factor-induced proliferation of cultures of human prostate biopsies', *Eur Urol* 33.3 (1998): 340–7

21. S Delos *et al.*, 'Testosterone metabolism in primary cultures of human prostate epithelial cells and fibroblasts', *J Steroid Biochem Mol Biol* 55.3–4 (1995): 375–83

22. *Br J Clin Pharmacol* 18 (1984): 461–2

23. J L Descotes *et al.*, 'Placebo-controlled evaluation of the efficacy and tolerability of Permixon in BPH after exclusion of placebo responders', *Clin Drug Invest* 5 (1995): 291–7

24. W Vahlensieck Jr *et al.*, 'Benigne prostatahyperplasie-behand lung mit sabalfrucht-estrakt', *Fortscr Med* 111.18 (1993): 323–6

25. G S Gerber, 'Saw palmetto (Serenoa repens) in men with lower urinary tract symptoms: effects on urodynamic parameters and voiding symptoms', *Urology* 51.6 (1998): 1003–7

26. J Kondas *et al.*, 'Sabal serrulata extract in the treatment of symptomatic BPH', *Int Urol Nephrol* 28.6 (1996): 767–72

27. D Bach, 'Medikamentose Langseitbehandlung der BPH. Ergebnisse einer prospektiven 3-Jahresstudie mit dem Sabal extrakt IDS 89', *Urologe* [B] 35 (1995): 178–83

28. J Braeckman *et al.*, 'Efficacy and safety of the extract of Serenoa repens in the treatment of BPH: an open multicentre

study', *Eu J Clin Res* 9 (1997): 47–57

29. J-C Carraro *et al.*, 'Comparison of phytotherapy (Permixon) with finasteride in the treatment of BPH: a randomised international study of 1098 patients', *Prostate* 29.4 (1996): 231–42

30. A M Semino *et al.*, 'Symptomatic treatment of benign hypertrophy of the prostate. Comparative study of prazosin and serenoa repens', *Arch Esp Urol* 45.3 (1992): 211–13

31. M Grasso *et al.*, 'Comparative effects of alfuzosin versus Serenoa repens in the treatment of symptomatic BPH', *Arch Esp Urol* 48.1 (1995): 97–103

Chapter 3

1. F C Lowe and J C Ku, 'Phytotherapy in treatment of BPH: a critical review', *Urology* 48 (1996): 12–20

2. T J Wilt, 'Beta-sitosterol for the treatment of BPH: a systematic review', *BJU Int* 83.9 (1999): 976–83

3. E Kvanta, 'Sterols in pollen' *Acta Chem. Scand.* 22 (1968): 2161–5

4. A C Buck *et al.*, 'Treatment of outflow tract obstruction due to benign prostatic hyperplasia with the pollen extract Cernilton', *Br J Urol* 66 (1990): 398–404

5. E W Rugendorff et al., 'Results of treatment with pollen extract (Cernilton N) in chronic prostatitis and prostatodynia', *British Journal of Urology* 71 (1993): 433–38.

6. A C Buck *et al.*, 'Treatment of chronic prostatitis and prostatodynia with pollen extract', *Br J Urol* 64 (1989): 496–9

7. E W Rugendorff *et al.*, 'Results of treatment with pollen extract in chronic prostatitis and prostatodynia', *British Journal of Urology* 71 (1993): 433–8.

8. G Loschen and L Ebeling, 'Hemmung der Arachidonsaure-Kaskade durch einen Extrakt aus Oggenpollen', *Arzneim. Forsch./ Drug Res* 41 (1991): 162–7

9. Tunn Abine and M Krieg, 'Alterations in the Intraprostatic hormonal Metabolism by the Pollen Extract Cernilton N' in *Benign Prostate Disease* (W Vahlensieck and G Rutishauser [eds]; NY: Thieme Medical Publishers, Inc.): 109–14

10. G Loschen and L Ebeling, 'Hemmung der Arachidonsaure-Kaskade durch einen Extrakt aus Oggenpollen', *Arzneim.-Forsch./Drug Res* 41 (1991): 162–7

11. F K Habib *et al.*, 'In vitro evaluation of the pollen extract, Cernitin T-60, in the regulation of prostate cell growth', *Br J Urol* 66 (1990): 393–7

12. A Lewenstein, *ProstatBrit Presentation* (London: RSM, May 27th 1992) ProstaBrit

13. T Lian *et al.*, 'Inhibition of steroid 5-alpha-reductase by specific aliphatic unsaturated fatty acids', *Biochem J* 285 (1992): 557–62

14. K F Klippel *et al.*, 'A multicentre, placebo-controlled, double-blind

clinical trial of beta-sitosterol for the treatment of BPH', *Br J Urol* 80.3 (1997): 427–32

15. R R Berges *et al.*, 'Randomised placebo-controlled, double-blind clinical trial of beta-sitosterol in patients with benign prostatic hyperplasia', *Lancet* 345 (1995): 1529–32

16. M Paubert-Braquet *et al.*, 'Effect of Pygeum africanum extract on A23187-stimulated production of lipoxygenase metabolites from human polymorphonuclear cells', *J Lipid Mediat Cell Signal* 9.3 (1994): 285–90

17. G Mathe *et al.*, 'A Pygeum africanum extract with so-called phyto-estrogenic action markedly reduces the volume of true and large prostatic hypertrophy', *Biomed Pharmacother* 49.7–8 (1995): 341–3

18. C Carani *et al.*, 'Urological and sexual evaluation of treatment of BPH using Pygeum africanum at high doses', *Arch Ital Urol Nefrol Androl* 63.3 (1991): 341–5

19. J Breza *et al.*, 'Efficacy and acceptability of Pygeum africanum extract in the treatment of BPH', *Curr Med Res Opin* 14.3 (1998): 127–39

20. T Krzeski *et al.*, 'Combined extracts of Urtica dioica and Pygeum africanum in the treatment of BPH: double-blind comparison of two doses', *Clin Ther* 15(6) (1993): 1011–20

21. M Schotter *et al.*, 'Lignans from the roots of Urtica dioica and their metabolites bind to SHBG', *Planta Med* 63.6 (1997):

529–32

22. T Hirano *et al.*, 'Effects of stinging nettle root extracts and their steroidal components on the Na+,K+-ATPase of BPH', *Planta Med* 60.1 (1994): 30–3

23. K Riehemann *et al.*, 'Plant extracts from stinging nettle (Urtica dioica), an antirheumatic remedy, inhibit the proinflammatory transcription factor NF-kappaB. *FEBS Lett* 442.1 (1999): 89–94

24. H J Schneider *et al.*, 'Treatment of BPH. Results of a treatment study with the phytogenic combination of Sabal extract and Urtica extract in urologic speciality practices', *Fortschr Med* 113.3 (1995): 37–40

25. Metzker M *et al.*, 'Wirksamkeit eines Sabal-Urtica-Kombination-spraparates bei der Behandlung der benignen BPH', *Urologe* [B] 36 (1996): 292–300

26. J Sokeland and J Albrecht, 'Combination of Sabal and Urtica extracts vs finasteride in BPH. Comparison of therapeutic effectiveness in a one year, double-blind study', *Urologe* A 36.4 (1997): 327–33

27. T Krzeski *et al.*, 'Combined extracts of Urtica dioica and Pygeum africanum in the treatment of BPH: double-blind comparison of two doses', *Clin Ther* 15(6) (1993): 1011–20

28. X Zhang *et al.*, 'Effect of the extracts of pumpkin seeds on the urodynamics of rabbits', *J Tongji Med Univ* 14.1 (1994): 235–8

29. A Jonas *et al.*, 'Cactus flower extracts may prove beneficial in

BPH due to inhibition of 5-alpha-reductase activity, aromatase activity and lipid peroxidation', *Urol Res* 26.4 (1998): 265–70

Chapter 4

1. J H Cummings and S A Bingham, 'Diet and the prevention of cancer', *BMJ* 317 (1998): 1636–40

2. R M Sharpe and N E Skakkebaek, 'Are oestrogens involved in falling sperm counts and disorders of the male reproductive tract?', *Lancet* 341 (1993): 1392–5

3. Giovannucci *et al.*, 'A prospective study of dietary fat and risk of prostate cancer', *J. Natl Cancer Inst* 85 (1993): 1571–9

4. R B Hayes *et al.*, 'Dietary factors and risks for prostate cancer among blacks and whites in the US', *Cancer Epidemiol Biomarkers Prev* 8.1 (1999): 25–34

5. L Denis *et al.*, 'Diet and its preventive role in prostatic disease', *Eur Urol* 35.5–6 (1999): 377–87

6. W B Grant, 'An ecologic study of dietary links to prostate cancer', *Altern Med Rev* 4.3 (1999): 162–9

7. H Adlercreutz *et al.*, 'Urinary excretion of lignans and isoflavonoid phytoestrogens in Japanese men and women consuming a traditional Japanese diet' *Am. J. Clin. Nutr.* 54.6 (1991): 1093–1100

8. H Adlercreutz *et al.*, 'Plasma Concentrations of phyto-oestrogens in Japanese men', *Lancet* 342 (1993): 1209–10

9. F Gu, 'Changes in the prevalence of BPH in China', *Chin Med J*

110.3 (1997): 163–6

10. J Geller *et al.*, 'Genistein inhibits the growth of human patient BPH and prostate cancer in histoculture', *Prostate* 34.2 (1998): 75–9

11. 'Diet, breast cancer and sex hormone metabolism'. *Am NY Acad Sci* 595 (1990): 281–90.

12. K Griffiths *et al.*, 'Phytoestrogens and diseases of the prostate gland', *Ballieres Clin Endocrinol Metab* 12.4 (1998): 625–47

13. E Giovannucci, 'Tomatoes, tomato-based products, lycopene and cancer: review of the epidemiologic literature', *J Natl Cancer Inst* 91.4 (1999): 317–31

14. P H Gann *et al.*, 'Lower prostate cancer risk in men with elevated plasma lycopene levels: results of a prospective analysis', *Cancer Res* 59.6 (1999): 1225–30

15. M Pastori *et al.*, 'Lycopene in association with alpha-tocopherol inhibits at physiological concentrations proliferation of prostate cancer cells', *Biochem Biophys Res Commun* 250.3 (1998): 582–5

16. A V Rao, 'Serum and tissue lycopene and biomarkers of oxidation in prostate cancer patients: a case control study', *Nutr Cancer* 33.2 (1999): 159–64.

17. La Vecchia *et al.*, 'Diet and cancer risk in northern Italy: an overview', *Tumori* 76.4 (1990): 306–10

18. O P Heinonen *et al.*, 'Prostate cancer and supplementation with alpha-tocopherol and beta-carotene: incidence and mortality in a

controlled trial', *J Natl Cancer Inst* 90.6 (1998): 440–6

19. Hunt *et al.*, 'Effects of dietary zinc depletion on seminal volume and zinc loss, serum testosterone concentrations and sperm morphology in young men', *Am J Clin Nutr.* 56 (1992): 148–57

20. Marma *et al.*, *Fertil Steril* 26 (1975): 1057

21. Vye Zaichick *et al.*, 'Zinc in the human prostate gland: normal, hyperplastic and cancerous', *Int Urol Nephrol* 29.5 (1997): 565–74

22. K Yoshizawa *et al.*, 'Study of prediagnostic selenium level in toe nails and the risk of advanced prostate cancer', *J Natl Cancer Inst* 90.16 (1998): 1219–24

23. D Feldman *et al.*, 'Vitamin D and prostate cancer', *Adv Exp Med Biol* 375 (1995): 53–63

24. H Matzkin and M S Soloway, 'Cigarette smoking: a review of possible associations with BPH and prostate cancer', *Prostate* 22.4 (1993): 277–90

25. E A Platz *et al.*, 'Alcohol consumption, cigarette smoking and risk of BPH', *Am J Epidemiol* 149.2 (1999): 106–15

26. E A Platz *et al.*, 'Physical activity and BPH', *Arch Intern Med* 158.12 (1998): 2349–56

Index

Thorsons
Directions for life